Contemporary Diagnosis and Management of the Patient With Epilepsy™

Second Edition 1996

By

Ilo E. Leppik, MD

Director of Research, MINCEP Epilepsy Care,
Minneapolis, Minnesota
and
Clinical Professor of Neurology and Pharmacy Practice,
University of Minnesota

Published by
Handbooks in Health Care, Newtown, Pennsylvania, USA

International Standard Book Number: 1-884065-05-8

Library of Congress Catalog Card Number: 95-79101

Table of Contents

This book has been prepared and is presented as a service to the medical community. The information provided reflects the knowledge, experience, and personal opinions of Ilo E. Leppik, MD, Clinical Professor of Neurology and Pharmacy Practice, University of Minnesota, and Director of Research, MINCEP Epilepsy Care, Minneapolis, Minnesota.

This book is not intended to replace or to be used as a substitute for the complete prescribing information prepared by each manufacturer for each drug. Because of possible variations in drug indications, in dosage information, in newly described toxicities, and in other items of importance, reference to such complete prescribing information is definitely recommended before any of the drugs discussed are used or prescribed.

Acknowledgments

I would like to extend my thanks in preparing this book to Matthew T. Corso of Handbooks in Health Care Co., for his editing of the copy, and to my wife, Peggy, and our children, Peter, David, and Karina, for their patience and support.

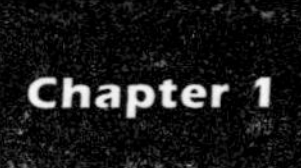

Chapter 1

Introduction

"Epilepsy is an illness of various shapes and horrible."—Aretaeus[1]

Epilepsy is a common neurologic disorder. For example, epidemiologic studies have shown that the cumulative adjusted lifetime incidence of epilepsy in Rochester, Minnesota, is 3.1% by age 80.[2] In other words, if all persons lived to age 80 in that community, 31 in 1,000 will have or have had a diagnosis of epilepsy sometime in their lives. This makes epilepsy the third most common neurologic disorder, following stroke and Alzheimer's disease.

Examples of the number of cases of epilepsy around the world are given in Table 1.[2] The number of *active cases* in any given year in most countries where valid prevalence statistics are available is 5 to 8 per 1,000 (or 0.5% to 0.8%). Preliminary statistics also show that epilepsy may be more common in some underdeveloped countries. The difference between the 3.1% by age 80 incidence and the 0.5%-to-0.8% range in any given year is explained by the fact that many patients outgrow their epilepsy. The 3.1% lifetime figure includes all persons who continue to experience epileptic seizures as well as those who experienced such seizures at some time in their lives but no longer do so.

Table 1
Active Cases of Epilepsy (prevalence) per 1,000[2]

Country	Age-Adjusted Prevalence
Iceland	3.7
England	4.4
Nigeria	5.0
India (Bombay)	3.6
Guam	6.1
Poland	8.1
USA	
• Rochester, Minnesota	6.0
• Copiah County, Mississippi	7.0

Epilepsy, by definition, is a condition in which an individual is predisposed to recurrent seizures because of a cen-

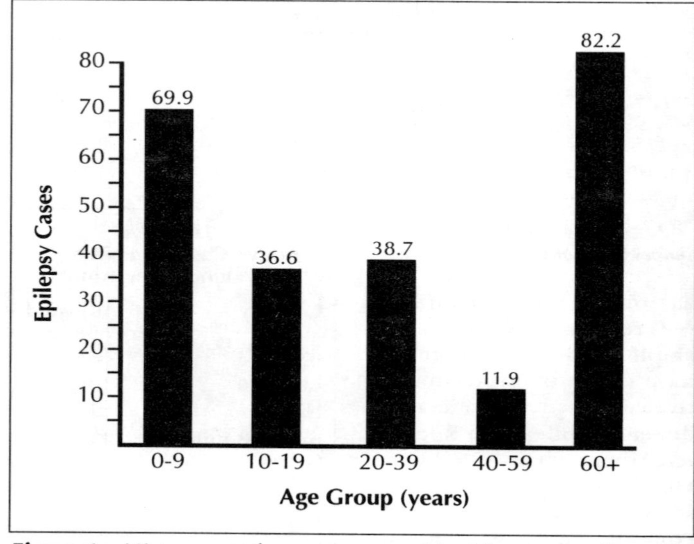

***Figure 1**—Histogram of average annual incidence of epilepsy by age; new cases per year per 100,000. Data from Rochester, Minnesota. Adapted from Hauser.[2]*

tral nervous system (CNS) disorder. A seizure is a sudden, involuntary, time-limited alteration in behavior, including a change in motor activity, in autonomic function, in consciousness, or in sensation, accompanied by an abnormal electrical discharge in the brain.[3]

Some studies have shown that the cumulative lifetime incidence of a person having a seizure from any cause is approximately 9%,[2] which is considerably higher than the cumulative lifetime incidence of epilepsy. Thus, many persons will have isolated seizures without ever developing epilepsy. This fact makes the evaluation and treatment of a person with a single seizure particularly challenging.

Many clinicians had believed that the onset of epilepsy is most common in children. But recent studies have shown that epilepsy's incidence is high among the elderly (Figure 1).[2] One survey of nursing home residents revealed that 10.1% (4,573 of

45,405) were receiving at least one antiepileptic drug.[4]

The causes of epilepsy are many; any disease that affects the central nervous system is capable of producing epilepsy. Yet, the most common cause remains that nettlesome category, "unknown." Thus, epilepsy is not a single disease, but rather a disorder with many causes. In the young, genetic syndromes and birth trauma are the most common causes. Cerebrovascular diseases are the most common causes of epilepsy in the elderly.

Epilepsy is also variable in its degree of severity. Some persons have mild epilepsy with seizures that are completely controlled with medicine. Others continue to have a few seizures, and some patients have intractable epilepsy with multiple seizures despite numerous treatments.

In addition, epilepsy is an episodic and paroxysmal condition. Most persons with epilepsy are completely normal between seizures, but are subject to unpredictable episodes of loss of consciousness and motor control. Thus, epilepsy is a frightening condition, misunderstood by many, including health-care professionals. This has placed an extra burden on the patient with epilepsy, who often faces discrimination in the workplace and in society.

Physicians caring for patients with epilepsy must not only have the medical knowledge to properly control seizures, but must also be sensitive to the impact this disorder has on the person as a whole. Simply controlling seizures without attending to the social and emotional issues will often lead to a less than ideal outcome.[3]

This handbook is intended to serve as an introduction to this fascinating disorder, which can so profoundly affect the mind, consciousness, and motion.

References

1. Temkin O: *The Falling Sickness: A History of Epilepsy from the Greeks to the Beginnings of Modern Neurology.* 2nd ed, revised. Baltimore and London, Johns Hopkins Press, 1971, pp 7-9.

2. Hauser WA, Hesdorffer DC: *Epilepsy: Frequency, Causes, and Consequences.* New York, Demos Publications, 1990, pp 1-51.

3. Gumnit RJ, Leppik IE: The epilepsies. In: Rosenberg R, ed. *Comprehensive Neurology.* New York, Raven Press, 1991, pp 311-336.

4. Cloyd JC, Lackner TE, Leppik IE: Drugs in the elderly: pharmacoepidemiology and pharmacokinetics. *Arch Fam Med* 1994;3:589-598.

Chapter 2

The Classification of Seizures

Over the ages, many different terms have been used to describe epilepsy and seizures. This proliferation of descriptive words has led to unnecessary confusion among patients and health-care providers when discussing the disorder. This chapter will review the terminology and classification of seizures; in Chapter 3 we will examine the classification of the epilepsies.

The word "seizure" is sometimes used vaguely to refer to a sudden, catastrophic event, especially if the precise nature of the event is unknown. Other words that have been used in this context are "fit," "spell," and "attack," among others. In this handbook, a seizure is defined as a paroxysmal, time-limited event that results from abnormal neuronal activity in the brain. However, physicians may face a situation in which the precise nature of the event being evaluated has not been determined. In this circumstance, "possible seizure" would be a better description to avoid labeling someone as epileptic before a definitive diagnosis is made.

Although many persons are familiar with the most dramatic form of seizures—the tonic-clonic or "grand mal" seizure—many behavioral patterns may occur as part of a seizure.

Behavioral Features

The major behavioral features of seizures that distinguish them from usual activity are that they are stereotypical and repetitive. They lack the typical modulation seen with volitional behavior. For example, a clonic seizure involves maximal contraction of one group of muscles, followed by relaxation, with the cycle usually repeated a few times per second. This very primitive movement pattern accomplishes no useful function and is in marked contrast to the usual complex, modulated activity that our muscle groups are capable of performing.

More common than the dramatic generalized tonic-clonic

Table 1
Epileptic Seizures: Classification and Characteristics, as Proposed by the ILAE[2]

I. Partial Seizures (Focal Seizures)

A. Simple partial seizures
  1. with motor signs
  2. with somatosensory or special sensory symptoms
  3. with autonomic symptoms
  4. with psychic symptoms

B. Complex partial seizures
  1. simple partial onset followed by impairment of consciousness
  2. with impairment of consciousness at the onset

C. Partial seizures evolving to secondarily generalized seizures
  1. simple partial seizures
     (a) evolving to generalized seizures
  2. complex partial seizures
     (b) evolving to generalized seizures
  3. simple partial seizures evolving to complex partial seizures evolving to generalized seizures

II. Generalized Seizures (Convulsive or Nonconvulsive)

A. 1. typical absence seizures (petit mal)
   2. atypical

B. Myoclonic seizures

C. Clonic seizures

D. Tonic seizures

E. Tonic-clonic seizures (grand mal)

F. Atonic seizures

III. Unclassified Epileptic Seizures

- Includes all those seizures that cannot be classified because of incomplete data or because they defy classification into the above catagories; for example, neonatal seizures with swimming movements.

IV. Status Epilepticus

Used with permission, *Epilepsia 1981;22:489-501.*

seizures (GTS) are the partial seizures. These may be simple or complex. In 1954, Penfield used the term "automatism" to describe the unconscious, meaningless behavior exhibited by persons having a complex partial seizure.[1] A patient with complex partial seizures may perform activities that superficially appear normal, but that are done without seeming comprehension of the social setting. For example, one of my patients was described by his friends as experiencing the following: while playing cards, he developed a blank look on his face, put down his cards, walked slowly to the refrigerator, opened its door, urinated, and then appeared confused. Upon recovering awareness, he had no recollection of this event. Fortunately, his friends were aware of his epilepsy, and had seen other episodes of his unusual behavior.

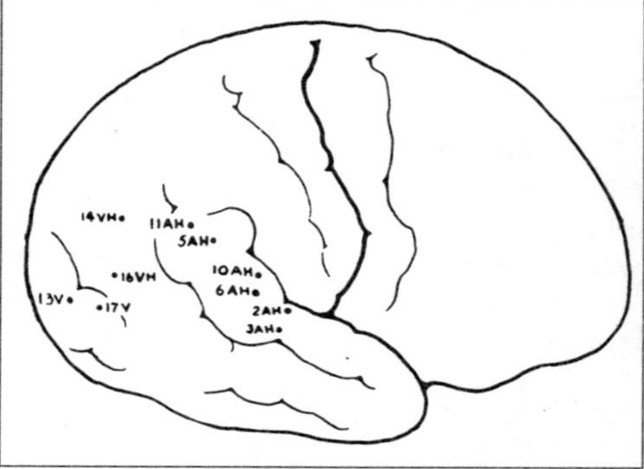

Figure 1—*Classic depiction of partial stimulation record. V=visual response; VH=visual hallucinatory seizure; AH=auditory hallucinatory seizure. Reprinted with permission from* Epilepsy and the Functional Anatomy of the Human Brain. 1st ed. Boston, Little, Brown and Co, 1954, p 464.

One of the major developments in epileptology of the last few decades has been the adoption of the International Classification of Epileptic Seizures (ICES).[2] At the core of this scheme, illustrated in Table 1, is the recognition of two major categories of seizures: those that begin locally in a specific region of the brain and then spread (partial seizures), and those that are generalized at onset (generalized seizures). Much of the basis for this classification is the recognition that the brain is highly organized, with specific functions represented in discrete anatomical regions. Thus, epileptic seizures that have their genesis in a discrete region of the brain (focus) are classified as partial seizures (Table 1). Conversely, those seizures for which there is no identifiable focal origin are classified as generalized. This division by physiologic criteria has proven useful in understanding epilepsy and in determining therapeutic strategies. This concept was elegantly discussed in a seminal book, *Epilepsy and the Functional Anatomy of the Human Brain,* by Penfield and Jasper.[1] This work was important in our understanding of the brain's organization (Figure 1). Their book provides numerous case reports of patients who had epilepsy surgery under local anesthesia, and those patients' responses to direct cortical stimulation. This stimulation was done both to identify the function of the cortex, which might need to be surgically removed, and relate it to the focus or site of onset of a patient's seizure.

In addition to clinical features, the electroencephalograph (EEG) is essential in classifying seizures: partial seizures have focal discharges, while generalized seizures have abnormalities over all head regions at onset (Table 2).

Simple Partial Seizures

The partial seizures are further subdivided by their effect on consciousness. Seizures in which consciousness is not altered are termed simple. An example of a simple partial sei-

Table 2
Summary of Clinical and EEG Features of Seizures

Seizure	Usual Duration	Loss of Consciousness	Postseizure Confusion	EEG During Seizure
Simple partial	5-10 sec	no	no	normal or focal spikes
Complex partial	variable; 5-10 sec, 1-2 min, 5+ min rarely	yes	yes	focal activity spreading to involve one or both hemispheres
Absence	5-10 sec, may cluster	yes	no	generalized, 3 per second, spike and wave
Generalized tonic-clonic	1-2 min	yes	yes	series of generalized, high-amplitude spikes

zure is a feeling such as that of a breeze over an extremity. "Aura" is the original Greek word for breeze, and was described in the medical writings of Hippocrates as the first sensation felt by a young man just before he was stricken with a generalized tonic-clonic seizure.[3] We now know that the origin of this kind of seizure is in the somatosensory area of the brain, contralateral to the limb experiencing the feeling. This simple partial seizure may progress into a secondarily generalized tonic-clonic seizure. Using the old terminology, this patient would be described as having an aura, followed by a grand mal seizure. The Jacksonian seizure is one in which a patient has clonic activity, usually involving the hand, contralateral to a lesion in the motor cortex. This activity usually progresses to a generalized tonic-clonic seizure.

The only difference between a Jacksonian seizure and a grand mal seizure preceded by a sensory aura is the location of the focus, but this similarity is not easily deduced from the old terminology. Furthermore, seizure manifestations change with medical treatment, so that often a person with Jacksonian seizures may no longer experience generalized tonic-clonic seizures with treatment, but still have brief motor seizures or "minor motor" seizures by the old classification system.

Simple motor seizures (**I.** A.1. in Table 1) arise from the motor cortex (frontal lobe). Other simple motor seizures are those with versive or postural movements. Simple partial seizures may have somatosensory phenomena (feeling of a breeze), visual (light flashes, formed visual hallucinations), auditory (buzzing), olfactory, gustatory, and vertiginous symptoms. Autonomic symptoms include epigastric rising sensation (described by some as the feeling one gets going down a roller coaster), sweating, flushing, piloerection, and pupillary dilatation. Psychic symptoms include fear, anger, dreamy states, déjà vu, and visual distortions such as macropsia (things appear large).

These events are sometimes difficult to separate from psychological phenomena. The two key features of epileptic seizures that distinguish them from the manifestations of psychiatric disorders are that seizures occur paroxysmally, that is, without warning and without preceding provocative events, and that they occur in patients who are relatively free of significant psychiatric disorders. Also of help is the fact that most simple partial seizures last only a few seconds (Table 2). However, these distinctions can lose some of their diagnostic effectiveness when a patient suffering from a psychiatric disorder also has epilepsy.

Complex Partial Seizures

Complex partial seizures involve impairment of consciousness. This implies alteration of functioning in the mesial temporal lobes, in the orbitofrontal lobes, or in more widespread areas of the brain.

Complex partial seizures in the past have been referred to as psychomotor seizures, but this term is now considered vague and ill-defined. They have been called temporal lobe seizures, but we now know that they can originate from extratemporal structures. Loss or alteration of consciousness in epilepsy does not refer to coma; rather, a lack of understanding and memory of the event is implied. As Penfield[1] explained: "The state in which an individual is able to move about in a relatively normal manner but is, at the same time, suddenly lacking in understanding is called automatism. Subsequently, he will have amnesia for the period. He may seem to be an automaton and yet is sometimes partially receptive of direction from others."

Complex partial seizures may last a few seconds. These brief episodes may be confused with absence seizures, and not infrequently may be called "petit mal." In the past, some referred to these as temporal lobe absence seizures. However, a clear distinction must be made because medications used for absence seizures are not effective for complex partial seizures. Most complex partial seizures last for 1 to 3 minutes, sometimes longer. The patient usually experiences a period of confusion after the seizure, lasting for a few minutes. Patients cannot recall any of the events that occurred during the seizure.

The automatism has no lateralizing value. For example, one right-handed patient snapped his fingers during an automatism, yet his focus was in the right temporal lobe. Sometimes complicated behaviors occur during a complex partial seizure. These often involve partial undressing, urination, or other socially embarrassing behavior, of which the patient with epilepsy has no recall after the seizure. "Cursive epilepsy," characterized by frantic running, and "gelastic epilepsy," characterized by uncontrollable laughing, are complex seizures of posterior temporal origin and are classified under **I.** B.1. or **I.** B.2. (Table 1), depending on onset.

Any partial seizure can generalize into a tonic-clonic seizure. Indeed, patients with partial seizures rarely present initially to the medical system for their partial seizures. Instead, they are often brought to the hospital emergency department after an unrecognized and untreated partial seizure generalizes and the patient experiences a "grand mal" seizure. This is really a partial seizure with secondary generalization and implies a discrete focus.

Generalized Seizures

Generalized seizures can be convulsive, that is, tonic-clonic (grand mal), or nonconvulsive. Absence seizures are what many have called "petit mal" in the past. In medieval France, the term "grand mal," literally translated as the big sickness, was used to designate a great epileptic attack. In contrast, the term "petit mal" or little sickness was used to describe a small seizure.

Absence seizures are most common in childhood. They are manifested by impairment of consciousness, eye blinking, staring, and other minor facial movements. They last from a few seconds to a minute. However, they may occur many times a day in rapid succession. An important consequence is the time lost, with the result that many children often have poor school performance. (These are described in more detail in Chapter 3.)

Myoclonic seizures consist of quick muscle jerks. These may be bilateral or unilateral and are usually seen in specific epilepsy syndromes. Consciousness is not usually impaired. However, myoclonic activity may also be associated with other neurologic disorders (Creutzfeldt-Jakob disease, anoxia). Furthermore, it may be difficult to readily categorize myoclonus.

Tonic seizures consist of tonic spasms of truncal and facial muscles associated with flexion of upper extremities and extension of lower extremities. They are most common in childhood and may result in falls.

Clonic seizures are most common in children, and may resemble myoclonus except that there is a loss of consciousness and that the repetition rate is slower than in myoclonus.

Tonic-clonic seizures are the most dramatic of all seizure

types. Generalized tonic-clonic seizures begin suddenly, without warning. (If the patient reports an "aura," the event was most likely a partial seizure with secondary generalization). Typically, the patient cries out as tonic contraction of the trunk muscles forces expiration. The generalized tonic phase then becomes interrupted by short periods of relaxation followed by tonic contractions. Then, the periods of relaxation become more frequent and the clonic phase begins. The seizure is accompanied by a marked increase in heart rate and blood pressure. The seizures last 1 to 2 minutes. Occasionally, they may occur in rapid succession and become status epilepticus. After the seizure is over, incontinence may occur as the sphincter muscles relax. Not all tonic-clonic seizures are followed by incontinence. Full consciousness might not return for 10 to 15 minutes, and confusion and fatigue may persist for hours or days.

Atonic seizures are characterized by the patient suddenly dropping to the floor from a loss of tone in postural muscles. Atonic seizures are most commonly seen in children with the Lennox-Gastaut syndrome. The attacks generally last only a few seconds and can occur without any loss of consciousness. However, these seizures are dangerous because they have a high rate of injury from falls. It is often difficult to distinguish between atonic and tonic seizures.

References

1. Penfield W, Jasper H: *Epilepsy and the Functional Anatomy of the Human Brain.* Boston, Little, Brown and Co, 1954, p 27.

2. Commission on Classification and Terminology of the International League Against Epilepsy. Proposal for revised clinical and electroencephalographic classification of epileptic seizures. *Epilepsia* 1981; 22:489-501.

3. Temkin O: *The Falling Sickness: A History of Epilepsy from the Greeks to the Beginnings of Modern Neurology.* 2nd ed. revised. Baltimore and London, Johns Hopkins Press, 1971, pp 28-50.

Selected Reading

Engel J Jr: *Seizures and Epilepsy.* Philadelphia, FA Davis Co, 1989.

Chapter 3

Epilepsy and the Epileptic Syndromes

Epilepsy is a disorder of the central nervous system (CNS) whose symptoms are seizures. The clinician must try to determine the underlying epileptic syndrome because this has profound implications for treatment and prognosis.[1] In other words, the seizure is a nonspecific symptom of a disorder that must be further diagnosed. This is analogous to fever being the symptom of any number of disease processes. To help organize the diagnosis of the underlying disorder, the International League Against Epilepsy (ILAE) has developed a classification of the epilepsies and epileptic syndromes (Table 1),[2] which must be used in conjunction with the classification of seizures. Many of these syndromes have age-specific onset and clinical characteristics that have been clearly delineated (Table 2).

An epilepsy syndrome may include more than one seizure type. For example, a patient can have both simple partial motor and secondarily generalized tonic-clonic seizures (types **I.** A.1. and **I.**C. as listed in Table 1, Chapter 2), but only one syndrome (case 1 at end of this chapter). Or, a person with the syndrome of juvenile myoclonic epilepsy has absence, myoclonic, and generalized tonic-clonic seizures (types **II.** A.1., **II.** B., and **II.** E.). Consequently, physicians must consider a number of factors when attempting to identify a patient's epileptic syndrome (Table 3).

In the ILAE's classification system of the epilepsies, the primary distinction is based on the patient's seizure type, either partial or generalized. Thus, the fundamental distinction is between the localization-related versus the generalized epilepsies. Localization-related epileptic syndromes are often caused by identifiable lesions.

Many causes of epilepsy have been identified. Epilepsies associated with a brain disease or lesion are labeled secondary or symptomatic. Epilepsies occurring without identifiable cause are labeled primary or idiopathic. Inherent in a classification of primary and secondary epilepsies is the notion that some of the primary, currently idiopathic epilepsies have strong genetic foundations.[2] Idiopathic or primary forms of the various epilepsies usually carry a better prognosis than disorders that are caused by identifiable brain diseases.

The proper classification of seizures is of great value in helping localize the brain regions involved. But identifying the correct type of seizure is not necessarily useful in determining the underlying pathology. For example, when evaluating a patient with simple partial motor seizures involving the left hand, the clinician can deduce that there is a lesion in the right motor cortex hand area. However, one cannot determine if the lesion is a tumor, an arteriovenous malformation, cysticercosis, or a cerebral cicatrix (scar) from an old injury. Other studies are needed to determine the pathology, but knowledge of the site can help guide diagnostic studies.

Localization-Related (Focal, Local, Partial) Epilepsies (1)

Localization-related epilepsies are described as either idiopathic or symptomatic. In the idiopathic (genetic) category, only two specific syndromes have been identified, both appearing in childhood and both with specific clinical and EEG features. On the other hand, there are numerous symptomatic epilepsies.

Idiopathic (1.1)

Benign childhood epilepsy with centrotemporal spikes (Rolandic epilepsy) is a common syndrome, and may account for as many as one quarter of epilepsies in school-aged children.[4] It has its onset between ages 3 and 13. The seizures have a simple partial onset, usually beginning in the face and variably generalizing to tonic-clonic seizures. The seizures occur almost always at night.[5] The children have normal neurological examinations and no associated illnesses. The EEG findings are classic and consist of high-amplitude spikes and sharp waves in the central region, which are most frequent during light sleep. The EEG findings are so diagnostic that many pediatric neurologists feel that structural studies such as magnetic resonance imaging (MRI) are unnecessary. Etiology is genetic, with an autosomal dominant inheritance reported for the EEG trait, but less than 25% of patients with the EEG pattern ac-

Table 1
International Classification of Epilepsies and Epileptic Syndromes

1. Localization-Related (Focal, Local, Partial) Epilepsies and Syndromes

1.1 Idiopathic with age-related onset

At present, two syndromes are established, but more may be identified in the future:

- Benign childhood epilepsy with centrotemporal spikes
- Childhood epilepsy with occipital paroxysms

1.2 Symptomatic

This category comprises syndromes of great individual variability, which will mainly be based on anatomical localization, clinical features, seizure types, and etiological factors (if known).

2. Generalized Epilepsies and Syndromes

2.1 Idiopathic, with age-related onset, listed in order of age

- Benign neonatal familial convulsions
- Benign neonatal convulsions
- Benign myoclonic epilepsy in infancy
- Childhood absence epilepsy (pyknolepsy)
- Juvenile absence epilepsy
- Juvenile myoclonic epilepsy (impulsive petit mal)
- Epilepsy with grand mal seizures on awakening

Other generalized idiopathic epilepsies, if they do not belong to one of the above syndromes, can still be classified as generalized idiopathic epilepsies.

2.2 Idiopathic and/or symptomatic, in order of age of appearance

- West's syndrome (infantile spasms)
- Lennox-Gastaut syndrome
- Epilepsy with myoclonic-astatic seizures
- Epilepsy with myoclonic absences

tually develop seizures.[6] Prognosis is excellent; seizures are easily controlled with carbamazepine or phenytoin and almost all children outgrow these without sequelae by age 15.[7]

The syndrome of childhood epilepsy with occipital spikes is much less common; it is characterized by daytime seizures consisting of visual experiences followed by complex partial seizures. After the seizure, patients often have a headache. The EEG shows bilateral, high-amplitude spike-and-wave discharges in the occipital re-

2.3 Symptomatic
  2.3.1 Nonspecific etiology
    - Early myoclonic encephalopathy
  2.3.2 Specific syndromes
    - Epileptic seizures may complicate many disease states.
    - Included under this heading are those diseases in which seizures are a presenting or predominant feature.

3. Epilepsies and Syndromes Undetermined as to Whether They Are Focal or Generalized

3.1 With both generalized and focal seizures
- Neonatal seizures
- Severe myoclonic epilepsy in infancy
- Epilepsy with continuous spike waves during slow wave sleep
- Acquired epileptic aphasia (Landau-Kleffner syndrome)

3.2 Without unequivocal generalized or focal features
This heading covers all cases where clinical and EEG findings do not permit classification as clearly generalized or localization-related, such as in many cases of sleep grand mal.

4. Special Syndromes

4.1 Situation-related seizures
- Febrile convulsions
- Seizures related to other identifiable situations such as stress, hormonal changes, drugs, alcohol, or sleep deprivation

4.2 Isolated, apparently unprovoked epileptic events

4.3 Epilepsies characterized by specific modes of seizure precipitation

4.4 Chronic progressive epilepsia partialis continua of childhood

Used with permission, *Epilepsia 1989;30:389-399.*

gion; the course is benign.

Symptomatic (1.2)

Symptomatic localization-related epilepsies are the most common syndrome in adults and have many specific identifiable causes (Table 4). Despite the large number of causes in this category, seizure types are limited to partial seizures that often, if untreated, progress to secondarily generalized tonic-clonic seizures. Thus, the phenomenology of the seizure is helpful in directing attention to the fact that identifiable and potentially

Table 2
Pediatric Epilepsy Syndromes by Age of Onset

Newborns
- Benign neonatal convulsions (Fifth-day fits)
- Familial benign neonatal convulsions
- Early myoclonic encephalopathy
- Severe idiopathic status epilepticus
- Early infantile epileptic encephalopathy with suppression-burst

Infants
- Febrile convulsions
- West's syndrome: Infantile spasms
- Benign myoclonic epilepsy in infants
- Severe myoclonic epilepsy in infants
- Myoclonic epilepsy (myoclonic status) in nonprogressive encephalopathies
- Epileptic seizures caused by inborn errors of metabolism
- Myoclonic-astatic epilepsy of early childhood
- Lennox-Gastaut syndrome

Children
- Childhood absence epilepsy (pyknolepsy)
- Epilepsy with myoclonic absences
- Epilepsy with generalized convulsive seizures
- Benign partial epilepsies
- Benign epilepsy with centrotemporal (rolandic) spikes (BERS)
- Benign psychomotor epilepsy

treatable pathology is present, but is not helpful in identifying the etiology, which must be done by the diagnostic evaluation. The underlying pathology may be diffuse or multifocal, such as anoxia, physical trauma (head injury), or infections. Other causes are more focal, such as cerebrovascular disease (stroke, arteriovenous malformations, subarachnoid hemorrhage, venous thrombosis), brain tumors (astrocytomas, meningiomas, glioblastomas, metastatic tumors), and mesial temporal sclerosis. Mesial temporal sclerosis may be one of the most surgically treatable of the epilepsies and will be discussed more fully in Chapter 13.

However, despite careful history-taking and the use of improved diagnostic techniques, in many cases the

- Benign epilepsy with occipital spike-waves (BEOSW)
- Other benign partial epilepsies
- Benign partial epilepsy with extreme somatosensory-evoked potentials
- Landau-Kleffner syndrome
- Epilepsy with continuous spikes and waves during sleep
- Epilepsy with photosensitivity
- Eyelid myoclonia absences
- Self-Induced epilepsy

Older Children and Adolescents (Juveniles)

- Juvenile absence epilepsy
- Juvenile myoclonic epilepsy (JME)
- Epilepsy with grand mal on awakening (GMA)
- Benign partial seizures of adolescence
- Kojewnikoff's syndrome
- Progressive myoclonus epilepsies
  - Juvenile Gaucher's
  - Juvenile neuronal ceroid lipofuscinosis (NCL)
  - Lafora's body disease
- Unverricht-Lundborg disease (Finnish or Baltic myoclonus epilepsy)
  - Cherry-red spot myoclonus (neuraminidase deficiency)
  - Dyssynergia cerebellaris myoclonica (Ramsay Hunt syndrome)
  - Mitochondrial encephalopathy

cause of epilepsy cannot be determined. Consequently, epilepsy of undetermined origin is still the most common "syndrome" in this category.

Generalized Epilepsies and Syndromes (2)

The generalized epilepsies are most common in the pediatric population. Idiopathic (genetic) syndromes have been well defined in the last few years, and indeed, gene foci have been mapped for some, cementing firmly the concept of a specific identifiable syndrome.

Idiopathic with Age-Related Onset (2.1)

Benign neonatal familial convulsions is a relatively rare syndrome characterized by generalized seizures occurring only during the first week of

Table 3
Factors to Identify the Epileptic Syndrome

- Seizure type(s)
- EEG (ictal and interictal)
- Etiology
- Response to AEDs
- Inheritance
- Natural history

life. It must be differentiated from the long list of more serious symptomatic neonatal seizures. There is usually a clear family history and the seizures remit spontaneously after a few days. Gene mapping has identified a locus on chromosome 20 associated with this syndrome.[8] Another infrequent disorder, benign myoclonic epilepsy in infancy, is differentiated in this age group by an EEG with bursts of spike-and-wave discharges superimposed on an otherwise normal background.

Childhood Absence (Pyknolepsy) was referred to as "petit mal epilepsy" in the past. However, because of the wide misuse of the term petit mal, the more accurate term of childhood absence has been applied to this condition. The term pyknolepsy (pyknos refers to crowding) is also used to describe this condition[9] because seizures have a tendency to occur many times an hour. They consist of the typical absence seizures described in Chapter 2. Although each seizure may be short, the fact that these seizures occur in rapid succession often leads to considerable dysfunction because of the time the child loses from school and other learning activities. The EEG is characterized by the classical 3-per-second spike-and-wave discharge occurring on an otherwise normal background.[10] Structural studies are usually not indicated. Childhood absence epilepsy occurs in 2% to 4% of children with epilepsy. The major differential diagnosis of this staring behavior is brief partial complex seizures.

Childhood absence epilepsy remits in 40% of patients, so lifelong therapy may not be needed.[3] The two drugs that are most effective in absence epilepsy are ethosuximide and valproate. Because childhood absence epilepsy is benign, ethosuximide is recommended first; valproate is recommended when ethosuximide is insufficient or when the patient also has generalized tonic-clonic seizures. However, some may have generalized tonic-clonic seizures that persist into later life. There is a strong genetic predisposition, although a specific gene locus has not yet been mapped.

Juvenile myoclonic epilepsy (JME) has its onset during the teenage years and is a characteristic syndrome consisting of a triad of seizures (myoclonic, absence, and generalized tonic-clonic). Myoclonic seizures usually occur in the morning and involve primarily the upper extremities. The most common complaint is clumsiness or jitters, which is exacerbated by stress and is often initially mistaken for adolescent behavior. Generalized tonic-clonic seizures develop, usually in the morning. Absence seizures may be relatively difficult to detect. Not all persons have all three seizure types, but the EEG characteristics along with the history are usually diagnostic. It is important to differentiate this syndrome from localization-related epilepsies because treatment is highly specific; re-

Table 4
Some Causes of Symptomatic Localization-Related Epilepsies

Vascular
- stroke
- infantile hemiplegia
- arteriovenous malformations
- Sturge-Weber syndrome
- aneurysms (subarachnoid hemorrhage)
- venous thrombosis
- hypertensive encephalopathy
- blood dyscrasias (sickle cell anemia)

Infectious
- abscess
- meningitis and encephalitis
- toxoplasmosis
- rubella
- Rasmussen's syndrome (presumed viral)
- cysticercosis

Tumors
- meningiomas
- gliomas
- hamartomas
- metastatic tumors

Degenerative
- Alzheimer's
- multiple sclerosis

Congenital
- heterotopias
- cortical dysplasias

Traumatic
- prenatal and perinatal injuries
- head injuries

sponse to carbamazepine or phenytoin is usually poor, while valproate is very effective. A specific gene locus on chromosome 6 has been proposed for this familial syndrome.[11]

Symptomatic and/or Idiopathic (2.2)

This group of generalized epilepsy consists of a mixed set of clinical syndromes. What unites them in the classification is that their clinical manifestations are similar. Some children in these groups have identifiable symptomatic causes, while in others the etiology is undetermined, or idiopathic. Unlike category 2.1 (Table 1), in which seizures occur in the setting of normal intelligence as the sole manifestation of the syndrome, in this group mental retardation is common.

Infantile spasms, also known as West's syndrome or salaam seizures, begin between the ages of 4 and 12 months. It is defined by a specific seizure type, a spasm that consists of flexion at the neck, waist, arms, and legs, with either abduction or adduction of the arms. These are quick, lasting only a second, hence the name "blitzkrampf," or lightning seizure. These may occur hundreds of times a day. Infants with this syndrome usually develop normally until spasms occur, at which point there is arrest of psychomotor development. Approximately two thirds of patients have an EEG pattern described as hypsarrhythmia and one third have focal abnormalities. The hypsarrhythmia pattern is a disorganized mixture of spikes and slow waves that are different in each hemisphere.

The prognosis in infantile spasms is related to the underlying brain disorder and to the therapy.[2] Patients with idiopathic infantile spasms who respond to optimal therapy have the best prognosis. Those with severe encephalopathic disorders have the worst. Among all patients with infantile spasms, 20% die before 5 years of age, and of the survivors between 75% and 93% are reported to be mentally retarded; up to 50% have epilepsy later in life, and half of these develop the Lennox-Gastaut syndrome.

Current therapy of infantile spasms is adrenocorticotropic hormone (ACTH) initiated within 1 month of the onset of spasms. This is associated with 5% mortality from complications of therapy, most often overwhelming infection.[13] When ACTH and steroids are ineffective, conventional anticonvulsants are used, most often a benzodiazepine such as clonazepam. Recently, vigabatrin has been reported to be particularly effective for control of seizures if West's syndrome is caused by tuberous sclerosis.

Lennox-Gastaut syndrome has been designated to represent a combination of seizures—axial tonic attacks, tonic-clonic seizures, atypical absence seizures, and atonic or so-called drop attacks—with mental subnormality and an EEG pattern of slow (< 2.5 Hz) spike and wave.[14,15] Onset is between 1 to 8 years. Lennox-Gastaut syndrome is typically difficult to treat. Valproate, benzodiazepines, and felbamate are most effective,[16] but some of the other drugs sometimes actually worsen the akinetic and atypical absence seizures.

Epilepsies, Undetermined as to Focal or Generalized (3)

In this category of epilepsies are a number of pediatric syndromes (Tables 1 and 2) whose clinical natures have not yet been fully elucidated. Some patients may experience a mixture of focal and generalized EEG patterns and clinical seizures. This group includes a number of cases of myoclonic epilepsy with mental retardation.

Special Syndromes (4)

This category is designed to encompass conditions in which seizures do not occur spontaneously, but rather are related to specific stimuli. Thus, these patients probably have some predisposing CNS dysfunction. However, unlike the epileptic syndromes described above, treatment for these special conditions often consists of avoiding the specific stimuli, or treating only at the time of provocation. Also in this group are patients who have isolated seizures and may simply have a low seizure threshold.

Situation-Related Seizures

Febrile seizures occur among children from 3 months of age to 5 years of age who have fever and no evidence of another cause. Although their reported incidence varies, in one large study these seizures occurred in 4.2% of black children and 3.5% of white children.[17] A family history of febrile seizures was present in 8% to 22% of parents and in 9% to 17% of siblings of the patient. This study found that offspring of febrile seizure patients had an 11% chance of having this kind of seizure.

Prospective population-based studies indicate that febrile seizures are relatively be-

Table 5
Factors in Febrile Seizures Associated With Increased Risk of Epilepsy at Age 7 Years[18]

- Family history of later epilepsy
- Preexisting neurologic abnormality
- Complex febrile seizure
  - > 15 minutes duration
  - > 1 febrile seizure per 24 h
- Focal febrile seizure

Used with permission, *Pediatrics 1978;61:720-727.*

nign.[18,19] Febrile seizures are not associated with an increased risk of mental retardation or of serious neurologic impairment. Overall, the chance of epilepsy after febrile seizures is small, with 3% developing epilepsy by 7 years of age and approximately 7% by 25 years of age.[17,19,20] Epilepsy is more likely to appear when certain risk factors are present (Table 5).

The risk of additional febrile seizures is related to the patient's age at the time of the first febrile seizure. Overall, the risk of recurrence is 34%, although it is higher in younger children. Among those patients who have their first febrile seizure before the age of 12 months, the chance of a second seizure is 50%. For this reason, some authorities recommend initiating treatment for children with febrile seizures who are less than 18 months old.[21]

Treatment is controversial; many pediatric neurologists do not recommend treating simple febrile seizeures. When phenobarbital is given, the doses should be sufficient to produce blood levels of 15 mg/L or more; side effects, mainly adverse behavior, are expected in up to 40% of patients. Slight cognitive side effects of phenobarbital also offset potential benefits.[22] European reports indicate that diazepam per rectum given when fever occurs may be effective;[23-25] a rectal product for U.S. use is being developed. Phenytoin and carbamazepine are not effective in preventing recurrent febrile seizures.

Case Reports

When treating a patient with epilepsy, it is important to classify not only the seizure type, but also the epilepsy syndrome. As the following case histories demonstrate, doing so leads to a specific treatment plan and prognostic information.

Case 1: The parents of an 8-year-old boy were aroused one night by noise from his bedroom. When they rushed to his room they saw the bedsheets awry and their son breathing deeply. He appeared to have bitten his tongue. In the emergency department he was mildly confused, afebrile, and had a lacerated tongue. He was admitted for observation, and an EEG the next day showed centrotemporal spikes. No further tests were done and he was discharged on no medications after discussion with his parents. However, a second nocturnal seizure occurred a year later and he was given medication. He was treated until age 12, when the medication was discontinued.

Seizure type: secondarily generalized tonic-clonic (**I.**C)

Epileptic syndrome: benign childhood epilepsy with centrotemporal spikes

Etiology: idiopathic

Prognosis: spontaneous remission with maturity

Case 2: A 36-year-old, right-handed construction worker had been suffering from pounding headaches, often brought on by exertion, for about 1 year. He also noticed that he did not seem to have the strength and coordination in his left hand that he was accustomed to having. Also, he occasionally found that his left hand would "jerk" for a few seconds. This became progressively worse, but he did not seek medical attention until he had a generalized tonic-clonic seizure at home. He was admitted to St. Paul-Ramsey Medical Center in St. Paul, Minnesota, for evaluation and treatment. This case was presented before MRI scanning was available. A routine CT scan showed a vascular lesion in the right frontal region extending to the motor area. A CT scan with contrast demonstrated this to be an arteriovenous malformation (AVM). He was initially treated with phenobarbital and phenytoin. Consideration was given to surgery, but it was deemed too risky because of the AVM's large size and its involvement of the motor area. He has been well controlled for the last 12 years in that he has not had any more generalized tonic-clonic seizures, but he continues to have periodic simple partial seizures. He also continues to have intermittent headaches and has had some mild decrease of function in the left hand.

Seizure types: simple partial seizures with motor symptoms (**I.** A.1) and secondarily generalized tonic-clonic seizures (**I.** C)

Epileptic syndrome: localization-related symptomatic (1.2)

Etiology: arteriovenous malformation

Prognosis: lifelong risk for seizures with possible worsening of motor dysfunction and intracerebral hemorrhage from AVM.

Case 3: A 28-year-old woman was shot in the occipital area and rendered unconscious. She recovered consciousness many hours later. The bullet had not penetrated her skull. Some months later she began to see "rainbows" lasting for 2 to 5 minutes. Also, she seemed to experience some loss of vision. These symptoms, which were similar to migrainous phenomena, were not followed by headaches, although she had intermittent neuralgic occipital pain.

A few months later she had a generalized tonic-clonic seizure. EEG revealed occipital spikes. A CT scan was unremarkable. Initial treatment was with phenytoin. This failed to completely control her partial seizures, so carbamazepine was added. The two drugs in combination effectively controlled her seizures. One year later she was admitted to the hospital emergency department with continuous convulsions. Her phenytoin and carbamazepine concentrations were in the therapeutic range. Video-EEG showed no epileptiform activity during the seizures. Counseling for post-stress syndrome was instituted because it was clear that she was suffering from nonepileptic seizures of psychogenic origin. About 2 years after onset, she stopped having simple partial seizures, and the dose of phenytoin was gradually reduced, and then eliminated. Then her dose of carbamazepine was reduced to obtain levels of 4 to 6 μg/mL. Over time, her seizure threshold increased, that is, her propensity to have seizures decreased.

Seizure types: simple partial seizures with sensory symptoms (**I.** A.2); secondarily generalized tonic-clonic seizures (**I.** C); and nonepileptic seizures.

Epileptic syndrome: localization-related, symptomatic, and nonepileptic psychogenic (1.2)

Etiology: posttraumatic (for epileptic) and stress (for nonepileptic)

Prognosis: improvement over time

Case 4: A 7-year-old girl had a sudden decline in school performance. Her teacher noted frequent episodes of staring and blinking. A physician, suspicious of absence seizures, ordered an EEG. This was normal until she began hyperventilating, which induced an absence seizure with 3-per-second spike-and-wave discharges. She was treated with ethosuximide. Her school performance returned to its normal level. When she reached 12 years of age, the medication was tapered, and then discontinued. EEG was normal both during rest and hyperventilation.

Seizure type: absence (**II.** A)
Epileptic syndrome: childhood absence epilepsy (2.1)
Etiology: idiopathic
Prognosis: remission

References

1. Leppik IE: Epileptic syndromes: Genetic, diagnostic, and therapeutic aspects: introductory remarks and symposium overview. *Epilepsia* 1990; 31(suppl 3):S1-S2.

2. Commission on Classification and Terminology of the International League Against Epilepsy: proposal for the classification of epilepsy and epileptic syndromes. *Epilepsia* 1989;30:389-399.

3. Delgado-Escueta AV, Treiman DM, Walsh GO: The treatable epilepsies. *N Engl J Med* 1983;308:1508-1514.

4. Cavazzutti GB: Epidemiology of different types of epilepsy in school-age children of Modena, Italy. *Epilepsia* 1980; 21:57-62.

5. Loisseau P, Beaussart M: The benign seizures of childhood with rolandic paroxysmal discharges. *Epilepsia* 1973; 14:381-389.

6. Bray PF, Wiser WC: Evidence for a genetic etiology of temporalcentral abnormalities in focal epilepsy. *N Engl J Med* 1964;271:926-933.

7. Beaussart M, Faou R: Evolution of epilepsy with rolandic paroxysmal foci, a study of 324 cases. *Epilepsia* 1978;19:337.

8. Leppert M, Anderson VE, Quattlebaum T, et al: Benign familial neonatal convulsions linked to genetic markers on chromosome 20. *Nature* 1988;337:647-648.

9. Dreifuss FE: The epilepsies: clinical implications of the international classification. *Epilepsia* 1990;31(suppl 3):S3-S10.

10. Penry JK, Porter RJ, Dreifuss FE: Simultaneous recording of absence seizures with video tape and electroencephalography: a study of 374 seizures in 48 patients. *Brain* 1975;98:427-440.

11. Greenberg DA, Delgado-Escueta AV, Maldonado HM, et al: Segregation analysis of juvenile myoclonic epilepsy. *Genet Epidemiol* 1988;5:81-94.

12. Kellaway P, Hrachovy RA, Frost JD, et al: Precise characterization and quantification of infantile spasms. *Ann Neurol* 1979;6:214-218.

13. Riikonen R, Donner M: ACTH therapy in infantile spasms, side effects. *Arch Dis Child* 1980;55:664-672.

14. Gastaut H, Roger J, Soulayrol R, et al: Childhood epileptic encephalopathy with diffuse slow spike-waves (otherwise known as "petit mal variant"). *Epilepsia* 1966;7:139-179.

15. Markland ON: Slow spike-wave activity in EEG and associated clinical features: often called Lennox or Lennox-Gastaut syndrome. *Neurology* 1977;27:746-757.

16. The Felbamate Study Group in Lennox-Gastaut syndrome. Efficacy of felbamate in childhood epileptic encephalopathy (Lennox-Gastaut syndrome). *N Engl J Med* 1993;328:29-33.

17. Nelson KB, Ellenberg JH: Predictors of epilepsy in children who have experienced febrile seizures. *N Engl J Med* 1976;295:1029-1033.

18. Nelson KB, Ellenberg JH: Prognosis in children with febrile seizures. *Pediatrics* 1978; 61:720-727.

19. Nelson KB: Can treatment of febrile seizures prevent subsequent epilepsy? In: *Febrile Seizures.* Nelson KB, Ellenberg JH, eds. New York, Raven Press, 1981, pp 143-146.

20. Annegers JF, Hauser WA, Shirts SB, et al: Factors prognostic of unprovoked seizures after febrile convulsions. *N Engl J Med* 1987;316:493-498.

21. Fishman MA: Febrile seizures: the treatment controversy. *J Pediatr* 1979;94:177-184.

22. Farwell JR, Young JL, Hirtz DG, et al: Phenobarbital for febrile seizures: effects on intelligence and seizure recurrence. *N Engl J Med* 1990;322: 364-369.

23. Augrell S, Berlin A, Ferngren H, et al: Plasma levels of diazepam after parenteral and rectal administration in children. *Epilepsia* 1975;16:277-283.

24. Kanto J: Plasma concentrations of diazepam and its metabolites after peroral, intramuscular and rectal administration. *Int J Clin Pharmacol* 1975;12:427-432.

25. Thorn I: Prevention of recurrent febrile seizures: intermittent prophylaxis with diazepam compared with continuous treatment with phenobarbital. In: *Febrile Seizures.* Nelson KB, Ellenberg JH, eds. New York, Raven Press, 1981, pp 119-126.

Chapter 4

Evaluation of a Seizure

The most difficult decision in evaluating a presumed seizure is determining if it was a seizure, or if it was another condition (Table 1). Not all events associated with loss of consciousness and abnormal body movements are seizures (as defined in Chapter 1). Events may be mistaken for seizures upon initial presentation, but must be differentiated from epileptic seizures because their treatment is different.

Table 1
Some Conditions That May Be Mistaken for Seizures

1. Syncope (see Table 4)
2. Nonepileptic seizures of psychogenic origin (pseudoseizures or psychogenic seizures)
3. Breath-holding spells
4. Paroxysmal REM sleep behavior
5. Panic attack

The second most difficult decision when evaluating a presumed seizure is determining if the seizure portends the development of epilepsy. Not every seizure develops into epilepsy. The cumulative lifetime incidence rate for having at least one seizure is almost 9%, but the cumulative lifetime incidence of epilepsy is approximately 3%,[1] which means that only one third of patients who have a seizure ever develop epilepsy. Approximately one third of the 9% lifetime rate consists of children with uncomplicated febrile seizures who have no further seizures later in life and are not considered to have epilepsy. Another one third are persons who have only a single, isolated seizure, or have seizures in the context of a specific medical illness. The remaining one third of persons will develop recurrent seizures and be diagnosed as having epilepsy.

Thus, the occurrence of a seizure does not necessarily imply the presence of epilepsy. But a single seizure may be the initial event heralding the onset of epilepsy. To make an accurate determination about the probability of further sei-

Table 2
Evaluation of a Single Seizure

History of the Event

1. Careful review of events occurring days before the seizure
2. Presence of any prodromal symptoms (auras)
3. Description of seizure and circumstantial evidence should be obtained from a reliable observer and witness
4. Postictal observations—time to recovery of normal function

Medical History

1. Febrile convulsions
2. Head injury
3. Cerebrovascular or cardiovascular disease
4. Cancer
5. Substance abuse
6. Infectious disease

Family History

1. Febrile convulsions
2. Epilepsy in siblings, parents, or close relatives
3. History of neurologic disorders

Social History

1. Travel
2. Occupation

Physical Examination

1. Injury pattern
2. Cardiovascular system
3. Skin

Neurologic Examination

1. Focal postictal deficits
2. Focal neurologic deficits after recovery
3. Neuropsychologic assessment

Laboratory Evaluation

1. EEG
2. Structural study, MRI preferable
3. Routine laboratory assessment
4. Toxicologic screen

zures, a sophisticated and detailed evaluation must be performed (Table 2).

History of the Event

Most seizures occur in the absence of trained observers. Moreover, many persons who witness a seizure for the first time are often too frightened or preoccupied with trying to help the stricken person to observe events carefully. It would be useful to know if a seizure began as a partial seizure that then generalized, or if it was generalized from the onset. But this determination about how a seizure originated is rarely based on first-hand observation. Most of the seizures that attract attention are generalized tonic-clonic seizures. Yet, most adults have localization-related epilepsy with partial seizures. Often, partial seizures are not recognized as significant events, and they may

Table 3
Some Common Causes of Provoked Seizures

1. Massive sleep deprivation
2. Excessive use of stimulants
3. Withdrawal from sedative drugs or alcohol
4. Substance abuse
5. High fever
6. Hypoglycemia
7. Electrolyte imbalance
8. Hypoxia

be present for some time before a secondarily generalized seizure occurs. For example, for months one of my patients had episodes of staring at the television and not responding to his wife before he eventually had a generalized tonic-clonic seizure that led to his hospital admission. Structural studies revealed a glioma, and, in retrospect, the staring spells were complex partial seizures.

Events occurring before the seizure must be reviewed. It is important to determine if the seizure was provoked or unprovoked. Unprovoked means that there was no specific disturbance of homeostasis and that the event was truly paroxysmal. Many things can provoke seizures. A common example is college students who experience seizures after extensive sleep deprivation and excessive use of stimulants when preparing for examinations. The most frequent examples of provoked seizures are febrile convulsions that occur only during a high fever. Provoked seizures are much less likely to be predictive of subsequent epilepsy. Table 3 is a list of events that may precipitate seizures but do not have a high association with the development of epilepsy.

Sometimes a patient, after fully recovering from the effect of the seizure, will recall prodromal symptoms. For example, the patient evaluated in case report 3 of Chapter 3 did not discuss the visual symptoms of seeing rainbows until after she had fully recovered from her generalized tonic-clonic seizure, and then only after she was asked if she had any unusual visual phenomena. The information pointing to focal neurologic involvement can be crucial in helping classify and, more importantly, localize, the onset of a seizure.

Epilepsy and Syncope

One of the physician's most important tasks in evaluating a patient with an episode of loss of consciousness is to determine if the event was a seizure or syncope.[2] Syncopal events are the most common symptoms confused with seizures,

Table 4
Differential Diagnosis of Syncope

1. Vasovagal attack
   - hyperventilation-induced syncope
2. Cardiac
   - atrioventricular block
   - Adams-Stokes attack
   - sinoatrial block
   - paroxysmal tachycardia
   - reflex cardiac arrhythmia
   - other cardiac causes of decreased cardiac output
3. Hypovolemia
4. Hypotension
5. Cerebrovascular ischemia
6. Micturition syncope

especially if there is inadequate history or observational data. There are many causes of syncope (Table 4). Brief clonic activity often accompanies syncope, and this can often lead to confusion regarding the diagnosis. However, the character of the muscle activity in syncope is mostly clonic or myoclonic, involves distal extremities, and rarely causes the classical axial tonic posturing seen in a tonic-clonic seizure. For example, a medical student, after donating blood and suffering from sleep deprivation, stood up, became pale, lost consciousness, fell slowly to the ground, exhibited some clonic activity of his hands, and lost bladder sphincter control. Although he was initially diagnosed as having had a seizure, the setting of the event and clinical features later led to the more accurate diagnosis of syncope. Table 5 lists those features that may help in differentiating syncope from seizures.

Loss of bowel and bladder sphincter tone occurs after a generalized tonic-clonic seizure but does not result in forceful evacuation of bowel or bladder contents. Rather, it is a passive emptying of the contents. Incontinence may also occur after any severe depression of consciousness. Cardiogenic syncope is seen most often in the elderly (Table 4). Micturition syncope and cough syncope[3,4] are reflex events leading to hypotension, loss of consciousness, falls, and sometimes injury. Cardiac causes of syncope must be considered, and can often be diagnosed by electrocardiogram (ECG).[5,6]

The terms psychogenic or pseudoseizure are being replaced by the more specific and less pejorative term, nonepileptic seizure. These events are often dramatic, with much motor activity that is usually considerably more complex than simple tonic-clonic activity. There may be pelvic thrusting, side-to-side head shaking, asynchronous extremity move-

Table 5
Clinical Features and Diagnostic Tests to Help Differentiate Generalized Tonic-Clonic Seizures and Syncope

Clinical finding	Seizure	Syncope
Injury*	common	rare
Urinary incontinence	common	rare
Confusion after event	common	rare
Headache	common	rare
Focal neurological findings	sometimes	never
Related to posture	no	often
Skin color	cyanotic	pale
Premonitory symptoms	short	long
Diagnostic tests		
Prolactin level	elevated	normal
Abnormal EEG	common	rare
Abnormal ECG	rare	sometimes

*The pattern of injury may be very helpful. Tongue or cheek biting is common with convulsions, rare with syncope. Some malingerers will bite the tip of the tongue, whereas with convulsions, usually only one side of the tongue is bitten by the molars. Persons with convulsions often fall forward or backward while the body is tonic or rigid, thus injuring the forehead, chin, or occipital area. Persons with syncope generally have gentler falls than persons with seizures.

ments, and other embellishments. Patients with these seizures, if properly diagnosed and treated, can have a favorable outcome. Thus, it is important to obtain as many details as possible surrounding the seizure.[7]

In the past, breath-holding spells in children were considered to be possible seizures. But they have clearly been shown to be nonepileptic and associated with behavioral problems. They may be associated with cyanosis or pallor.[8]

Medical History

A careful review of a patient's medical history is necessary. This may be impossible during or immediately after the seizure because the patient may be postictal, confused, disoriented, or unable or unwilling to disclose sensitive information, such as drug abuse. For example, a woman from the Twin Cities went to Arizona to visit relatives. A few days after arriving, she had two generalized tonic-clonic seizures in one day. She was told she had epilepsy and was started on antiepileptic medications. Upon returning, she was reevaluated, and only after a thorough review of events surrounding the seizure did she reveal that she had been a heavy user of benzodiazepines for sleep and anxiety, and had forgotten to take her medications to Arizona. In retrospect, she had seizures provoked by benzodiazepine withdrawal.

Because their parents never tell them, many persons do not know that they had febrile convulsions as children. Many families regard epilepsy as an embarrassment and often never reveal to the rest of the family the fact that a relative has had the disorder. Obviously, travel, work stress, sleep deprivation, and other factors may be important and must be fully evaluated.

Physical Examination

The first physician to evaluate the patient must perform a careful physical examination, directed toward finding specific signs that would help determine if the event was a seizure, and, if so, establishing its cause.

During a generalized tonic-clonic seizure, the CNS is in a state of maximal excitation, and all systems influenced by the brain are in a state of stimulation. Pulse rate increases, blood pressure rises, salivation increases, pupils dilate, and there is an excessive release of some hormones, such as prolactin. Respirations cease in the tonic phase and may be irregular in the clonic phase. The patient may appear frighteningly cyanotic in the tonic phase, but this color may be misleading because during the tonic phase intrathoracic pressure is increased and venous return is impeded, resulting in increased volume of desaturated blood in the face. After the seizure, there is respiratory and metabolic acidosis, and the response to this is marked increase in respiratory drive. Objects should not be placed in the patient's mouth because these may impede respiration and induce vomiting.

Vital Signs

After generalized tonic-clonic seizures, the pulse is usually strong and rapid. Depending on the patient's physical condition and age, tachycardia may persist for a few minutes or much longer. One of my patients once compared the physical exertion of a tonic-clonic seizure to running 1 mile. Although the seizure is usually only 1 or 2 minutes long, all major muscle groups are maximally contracted. This places considerable stress on the cardiovascular system, which is usually well tolerated by younger patients but may cause problems in the elderly. The presence of cardiac arrhythmias suggests that the seizure may have been related to a cardiogenic event resulting in cerebral hypoxia.

Respirations after a generalized tonic-clonic seizure are usually deep and rapid as the patient hyperventilates to overcome the respiratory acidosis, lactacidemia, and oxygen depletion. After syncope, respirations are usually normal. Patients who have had hyperventilation-induced syncope often experience slowed respiratory rate because of the hypocarbia. Airway patency must be evaluated. For example, a Minnesota Twins fan was treated for what were initially thought to be epileptic seizures during an exciting game. But it was quickly determined that his condition was the result of an aspirated hot dog leading to cerebral hypoxia.

Blood pressure is usually elevated for a few minutes after a generalized tonic-clonic seizure. Hypotension is unusual after a seizure, but its presence in the elderly may suggest the occurrence of a myocardial infarction.

After a single, generalized tonic-clonic seizure, body temperature is usually normal. The presence of fever raises the possibility of a reactive seizure, such as a benign febrile convulsion in children or an infection in adults.

General Appearance

Most patients are comatose, lethargic, or confused after a generalized tonic-clonic seizure. Hyperexcitability, aggression, or agitation are unusual and may suggest the patient's use of drugs or a psychological disorder.

HEENT

Examination of the head can be very informative. First, signs of new and old trauma must be assessed because injuries are common with a tonic-clonic seizure. The body becomes rigid, the patient loses consciousness, and falls either forward or backward, depending on the strengths of the muscle groups. With syncope, there is usually a prolonged prodromal period and the patient usually "slides" to the ground because consciousness is not abruptly lost. Scars can be important clues to past head injuries and intracranial surgery that may predispose a patient to seizures and epilepsy. Because patients with severe, intractable epilepsy have frequent falls either forward or backward, multiple scars with thickening of subcutaneous tissue develop on the chin, forehead, and occipital area. Injuries to the side of the head are much less common.

Tongue biting is a common consequence of a tonic-clonic seizure. Usually, one side of the tongue is bitten with the molars or incisors as the tongue is trapped by the tonic contraction of the masseter muscles. Occasionally, patients with nonepileptic seizures, knowing the importance of tongue biting, will intentionally bite the tip of their tongue to give the appearance of a seizure. These bites, however, are usually very shallow and do not bleed as profusely as the involuntary tongue bites with an epileptic seizure.

Teeth fractures may occur from falls associated with generalized tonic-clonic seizures, but are rare in other kinds of seizures.

Excessive salivation occurs from stimulation of the parotid glands and from tonic contraction of the masseter muscles that empty the contents into the oral cavity. This, coupled with rapid, deep respiration after the seizure, leads to the classical frothing at the mouth. This is not usually seen in patients with nonepileptic seizures but cases of malingerers using soap to imitate the frothing have been reported throughout history.[9]

Clear fluid that drains from the nose may indicate the leakage of cerebrospinal fluid from a fracture of the cribriform plate resulting from a skull fracture.

An asymmetrical head may be a clue to the presence of underlying injury to the brain in early childhood.

Careful examination of the eyes may reveal small neurofibromatoses of the iris as a clue to the presence of von Recklinghausen's disease. Funduscopic examination may show papilledema, a sign of increased intracranial pressure from tumor, pseudotumor cerebri, or recent intracerebral hemorrhage. The presence of optic atrophy, macular degeneration, "cherry red spot/mulberry" tumor (tuberous sclerosis), angiomatosis retinae of von Hippel-Lindau disease, and other anomalies open specific areas for differential diagnosis and need further evaluation.

A patient's dysmorphic facial features should be evaluated because they may provide clues to specific syndromes. For example, patients with Down syndrome may develop epilepsy in adulthood.

Table 6
The Neurocutaneous Syndromes (Phakomatoses)

All of these are characteristic syndromes with specific findings and are noted primarily for their tendency to be expressed in the skin and brain, although other organs may be involved. All but Sturge-Weber syndrome are inherited.

- Neurofibromatosis (von Recklinghausen's disease)
- Tuberous sclerosis
- von Hippel-Lindau disease
- Ataxia-telangiectasia (Louis-Bar's syndrome)
- Sturge-Weber syndrome (encephalofacial angiomatosis)

Neck

The neck must be examined for injuries. Fracture of the cervical spine may occur during a seizure-precipitated fall. Hyperthyroidism or parahyperthyroidism may be associated with seizures. Presence of carotid bruits should direct attention to cerebrovascular causes of seizures.

Lungs

Aspiration may occur in the postictal state, especially if vomiting has been induced by attempts to place tongue blades or other objects into the mouth. Pneumonia and other respiratory illness may be accompanied by seizures.

Heart

A thorough search should be made for cardiac disorders. It is not unusual to find patients treated for epilepsy who have a cardiac condition leading to cerebral hypoxia. In young adults, conduction defects may be present but overlooked. In the elderly, Adams-Stokes syndrome attacks, cardiac arrhythmias, and other conditions may be the etiologic factors (Table 4). The presence of a new myocardial infarction from the stress of a seizure must be excluded in the elderly patient.

Genitourinary

Loss of urine has been the hallmark of an epileptic attack since antiquity.[10] The Greeks knew that the loss of urine occurred after the tonic-clonic seizure. In fact, they considered the loss of urine and feces the seizure's terminal event, the body's expelling of the evil humors that were thought to cause the epilepsy. The release of urine is caused by relaxation of the sphincters in the postictal state and depends on the depth of coma after the seizure. In a patient with treated epilepsy, seizures are often less severe and not associated with loss of bowel or bladder sphincter tone. Thus, the absence of incontinence does not exclude the event from having been a seizure. Conversely, the presence of urinary incontinence does not establish the presence of a seizure. Some patients with profound syncope will experience incontinence, and some malingerers will deliberately soil themselves.

Extremities

Fractures and soft-tissue injuries may occur as a consequence of generalized tonic-clonic seizures. Burns may be seen in patients with complex partial seizures. Injuries are much less common from vasovagal syncope.

Unilateral smallness of hands and feet is seen in patients who have had early childhood brain injuries or intrauterine injuries. These may be unrecognized for many years and present as signs of epilepsy only later.

Skin

A number of neurocutaneous syndromes (phakomatoses, from the Greek "phakos," meaning birth mark) have specific manifestations (Table 6).[11] Neurofibromatosis is an autosomal-dominant disorder with variable clinical expression and occurs in 1 of 4,000 persons. The diagnostic criteria are six or more café au lait spots, two or more neurofibromas, and/or various combinations of bone dysplasias, optic glioma, or having a first-degree relative with the diagnosis. In tuberous sclerosis, the characteristic lesions are adenoma sebaceum (which should not be confused with acne) and hypopigmented skin areas. It is an autosomal-dominant condition affecting 1 in 30,000. Sturge-Weber syndrome consists of a facial nevus (port-wine stain) of the upper face often associated with ipsilateral intracranial calcifications. The cutaneous telangiectasia in Louis-Bar syndrome may be difficult to spot but are most common on exposed areas of skin.

Neurologic Examination

Mental Status. After the seizure, the postictal period (from the Greek "ictus," to seize) is an important time to search for clues that would help determine if the event was a seizure or another problem. Time to recovery of normal function is important (Table 5). Patients with syncope or nonepileptic seizures are usually lucid immediately after or within a few minutes of the event. Patients may be obviously confused for some time after a tonic-clonic seizure and, if carefully tested, found to have significant memory impairment for many hours and sometimes days. They may also have considerable retrograde amnesia for the event. One of my patients had been on a stressful trip, lost sleep, used alcohol, lost consciousness on his drive from the airport, and drove his car into a tree near his home. No one witnessed the event, but because he had lost bladder and bowel control, had bitten his tongue, and had been unconscious and far more confused than what would have been expected for this kind of accident, we concluded that he had had a provoked seizure.

Speech difficulties such as aphasia or anomia can be important clues to the lateralization of the onset of seizures. However, a patient's difficulty in speaking because of confusion or lingual injury from the seizure must be considered in the evaluation.

Cranial Nerves. Absence of the sense of smell may be caused by a fracture of the cribriform plate from recent or old head trauma.

Visual-field defect may be a prominent finding after a seizure if it had its onset in the occipital lobe. This can be of important lateralization value. The patient in case report 3 of Chapter 3 would often have an easily detectable scotoma (area of visual loss) for some hours after her seizure.

Asymmetrical pupils, especially a large unreactive one, suggest the presence of uncal herniation from a large intracranial mass such as an epidural hematoma. Small unreactive pupils may be associated with drug abuse.

Facial asymmetry may signify the presence of a stroke or, rarely, may be postictal.

Motor. Presence of postictal Todd's paralysis can be an important clue to help localize the brain region from which the seizure emanated. Weakness of one hand, for example, will point to the contralateral motor area. This information needs to be communicated to the radiologist so that specific views of the areas in question can be obtained.

Sensory. Unilateral sensory loss suggests an intracranial lesion in the contralateral parietal lobe.

Reflexes. Asymmetry of reflexes can be a useful clue to the hemisphere of origin of a seizure. The presence of a pathological reflex, such as Babinski's sign, may persist for hours after a seizure.

Laboratory Evaluation

Appropriate laboratory testing is essential in supplementing the patient's history and physical examination. The major tests are sampling of bodily fluids (blood, cerebrospinal fluid), imaging studies (x-ray, MRI), neurophysiologic studies (electroencephalogram), and functional tests (IQ testing, behavioral testing). Different sets of tests are needed, depending on the phase of the disorder. Acute evaluations are done as soon as possible after the initial seizure or onset of epilepsy; if the seizures develop into intractable epilepsy, more sophisticated evaluation is necessary to fully treat the patient for seizure control and for integration into society.

Blood

Glucose levels should be measured routinely in patients presenting to the emergency room with seizures of undetermined origin. In patients with epilepsy, blood glucose concentrations do not decrease significantly after generalized tonic-clonic seizures. However, both hypoglycemia and hyperglycemia can cause seizures.

In adults, blood glucose concentrations of less than 40 mg/dL may precipitate seizures. Seizures associated with hypoglycemia usually have a prodromal period characterized by weakness, confusion, and other symptoms, and the tonic-clonic phase may be associated with less vigorous motor activity.

Treatment with antiepileptic medication alone is ineffective, and not recognizing and treating the hypoglycemia may lead to CNS damage. Nonketotic hyperosmotic hyperglycemia may be characterized by both partial and generalized seizures. In these patients, blood glucose values of greater than 350 mg/dL are observed. Again, treatment of the underlying metabolic disturbance is essential. However, some patients with diabetes develop epilepsy from a lesion in the CNS. Poor control of diabetes may be associated with increased seizures, even without the extremes of blood glucose levels needed for hypoglycemic or hyperglycemic seizures. Phenytoin may affect release of insulin from the pancreas and thus may modify insulin requirements. The glucose tolerance test may be affected by phenytoin use.

In patients with epilepsy, carbamazepine may induce mild to moderate hyponatremia with sodium levels of 130 mEq/L or less. Most patients with mild hyponatremia associated with use of carbamazepine are not symptomatic, and the low sodium levels can be treated by water restriction. Severe hyponatremia, hypomagnesemia, and other electrolyte imbalances may cause seizures, but this is usually seen in the context of other illnesses.

Alcohol abuse is often associated with seizures. Usually, the seizures occur within 48 hours of the last drink and may be the brain's response to the withdrawal from alcohol. Blood alcohol levels may be low at the time of the seizure. A first seizure, even in the presence of alcohol use, should be fully evaluated, however, because sometimes the alcohol use triggers a seizure from CNS pathology. Also, some patients who abuse alcohol and have withdrawal seizures may eventually develop epilepsy, possibly from recurrent head trauma.

Drug abuse is another common cause of seizures, either from acute use or from withdrawal. Most drugs that are CNS stimulants can cause acute seizures. These include cocaine, amphetamines, PCP, and others. Measurable concentrations of these drugs may be found in blood or urine at the time of the seizure. Most sedative drugs such as barbiturates or benzodiazepines cause seizures only after withdrawal from chronic use, and measurable amounts of these may not be present in biological fluids at the time of the seizure.

A recent interesting development has been the finding that prolactin is elevated after epileptic seizures but not after nonepileptic psychogenic seizures.[12] The rise is usually dramatic, with levels increasing two to four times over baseline levels. However, the levels might not rise after partial seizures, and they may already be high from treatment with psychotropic drugs. Nevertheless, when one suspects nonepileptic seizures, a prolactin level should be obtained 15 to 30 minutes after the seizure is over.

A lumbar puncture should be done whenever CNS infection is suspected. However, after serial seizures, there may be a few white cells in the spinal fluid, findings that may suggest viral infections of the CNS. The minor pleocytosis from seizures is usually not enough to be confused with bacterial meningitis, which is accompanied by a few hundred or more white cells. Tubercular meningitis usually has elevated protein. Herpes encephalitis usually is accompanied by both white and red blood cells.

The most common cause of blood in the cerebrospinal fluid (CSF) is head trauma. In such injuries, the CSF may be clear or slightly pink and rarely grossly bloody, but microscopic examination reveals red blood cell (RBC) counts of 100 to several thousand per cubic mm. On the other hand, after subarachnoid hemorrhage, the CSF is grossly bloody, and the RBC count often exceeds 100,000/mm^3.

EEG

The electroencephalogram (EEG) is as vital to the diagnosis of seizures as is the ECG to cardiac disorders. The EEG was developed in the early part of this century and has played an important role in our understanding of epilepsy. One of its first successes was in identifying the classical 3-per-second spike-and-wave pattern characteristic of absence ("petit mal") seizure. Subsequent use of the EEG has confirmed its utility as a tool for diagnosing and classifying the epilepsies.

The background rhythm of a normal waking EEG consists of alpha activity of 20 to 50 μV (20 to 50 millionths of a volt). This activity is less than one hundreth of the amplitude of cardiac potentials. Thus, the EEG signals are much more difficult to detect, and with DC amplifiers, the EEG signals would be completely masked by muscle and cardiac activity. However, the development of AC amplifiers and bipolar recording has made it possible to measure the small, brain-generated potentials. But it should be obvious that in the presence of many relatively higher physiologic potentials, the EEG is subject to a great deal of artifact. Indeed, the most difficult aspect of EEG technology and interpretation is recognizing and excluding artifact.

Many mistakes have been made in diagnosing the presence of epilepsy when the abnormality later was determined to be artifact. Guidelines have been established for the proper technical qualifications for EEG laboratories and technicians, as have specialty boards for electroencephalographers.

An EEG requires the placement of 21 standard electrodes over the scalp. Additional electrodes, such as sphenoidal or nasopharyngeal, may be used in some laboratories if there is a question of complex partial seizures.[13] Care must be taken to apply electrodes properly, because movement of the contacts can generate potentials that may be much larger than the underlying EEG potentials. Also, because ECG artifact may be recorded easily, the use of a special channel to monitor the ECG is advisable so that these potentials can be recognized as cardiac in origin.

The EEG electrodes are connected to the amplifiers in pairs. These can be linked up into montages in a number of ways, and although there are general guides, many laboratories have developed their own specific configurations. Most EEG machines have at least eight channels, but 16 are preferred. These are recorded simultaneously because it is necessary to be able to develop a "map" of abnormal activity. In addition, since seizures may in some instances be triggered by hyperventilation or photic stimulation, these activation techniques should be performed in all EEGs.[13]

A major problem in the diagnosis of epilepsy is that the EEG may be normal for long periods relative to the time of the recording. Epileptiform

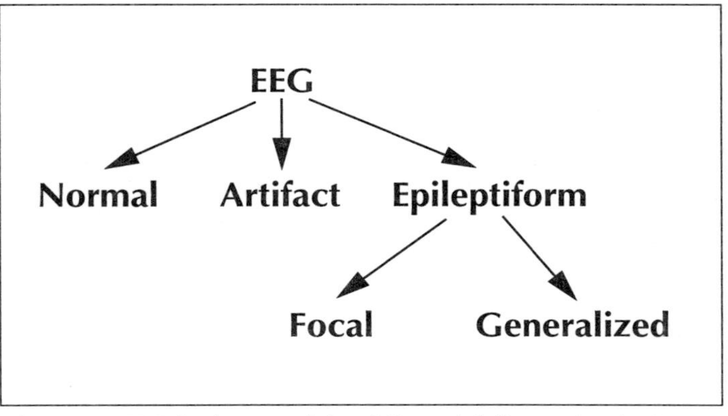

Figure 1*—EEG findings and the differential diagnosis of seizures. When the EEG contains epileptiform activity, the clinical diagnosis of epilepsy is secure and can be classified as localization-related (focal) or generalized. A normal EEG does not exclude the diagnosis of epilepsy. Artifact is troubling because it may be misinterpreted as epileptic, leading to an incorrect clinical diagnosis.*

A

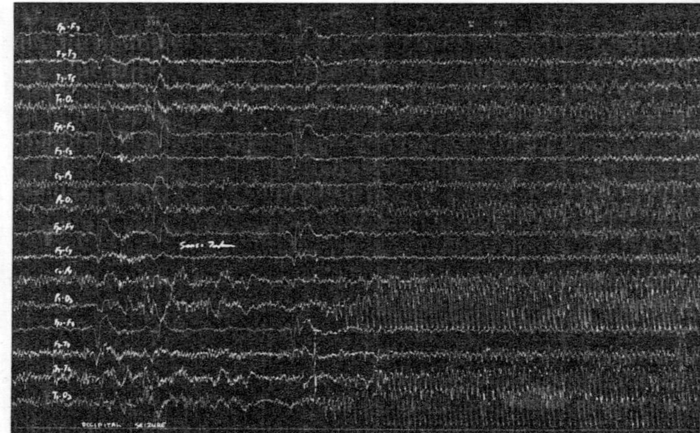

B

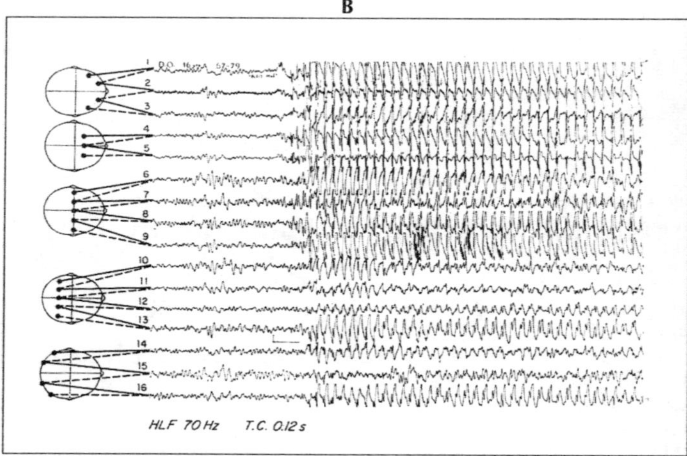

Figures 2A-2B—*Examples of EEG patterns. Figure A is from a patient with localization-related epilepsy. Seizures start at O_2 (electrode pairs P_2-O_2 and T_6-O_2) and spread to the left (T_5-O_1, P_1-O_1). All of the other high-amplitude activity is artifact. Figure B is from a patient with generalized epilepsy with absence seizures. (Courtesy of Fernando Torres, MD).*

activity is present only at brief intervals. Thus, it is not uncommon for a standard 30-minute recording to show no definite interictal activity in the presence of diagnosed epilepsy. Studies have shown that only 50% to 60% of routine EEGs (30 minutes, no sleep deprivation) obtained after a seizure in patients later clearly diagnosed as having epilepsy show epileptiform abnormalities. While normal EEGs are not useful, positive recordings are very helpful. Two things can be learned from the EEG. The first is the determination of the presence of epilepsy. The finding of an epileptiform EEG and the history of a seizure are strong evidence of the existence of a CNS disorder associated with a risk for further seizures. The second major purpose of the EEG is the classification of the epilepsy as localization-related or generalized. In addition, the localization of the discharge is helpful in determining the area of the brain containing the epileptogenic lesion (Figure 1). Knowledge of the probable site of origin can help guide other diagnostic studies.

The signature of an epileptic EEG abnormality is the sharp transient, which is usually a spike (less than 80 milliseconds) or a sharp wave (longer than a spike). A number of computer programs have been developed for spike detection, but for clinical diagnosis, visual interpretation is needed to screen out artifacts and place the occurrence of these sharp transients into clinical perspective. Spikes may be focal or generalized. Focal spikes are most often seen in the temporal regions. Muscle artifact, ECG potential, movement artifacts, and "electrode pops" must be differentiated from activity of CNS origin.

One of the most common errors made is the misreading of ECG potential or other sharp activity as spikes. In the intensive care unit, even the electromagnetic field generated by a drop of saline may be recorded and appear as a spike. In addition, there are cerebral potentials such as small sharp spikes, 14 and 6 spike and wave complexes, and other phenomena that have been misinterpreted as abnormal but now have been clearly established to be variants of normal activity occurring in some patients.[14] Some examples of EEG activity are shown in Figures 2A and 2B.

CT and MRI

Structural studies should be done in localization-related epilepsy, especially if the his-

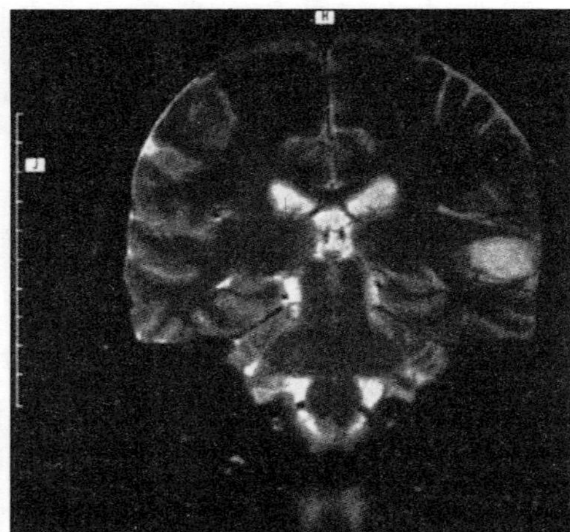

Figure 3—An MRI scan from a patient diagnosed with complex partial seizures from a glioma. A CT scan had been normal.

tory and clinical findings suggest the possibility of an intracranial lesion. In the past, CT scans were the diagnostic study of choice, but the MRI is now much more useful because of its better resolution. The CT scan is acceptable for determining the existence of vascular lesions and certain tumors larger than 1 cm, as well as regions of brain injury. However, low-grade gliomas that may be isodense with surrounding brain or subtle atrophy, especially in the temporal regions, may be missed with the CT scan.

Figure 3 is an MRI scan of a patient with a temporal lobe tumor that had not been clearly detected by a previous CT scan. Also, patients with mesial temporal sclerosis, who constitute a large fraction of patients with intractable epilepsy, may now be diagnosed by MRI. These "scars" of the mesial temporal lobe are rarely detected by CT scans. Yet, the detection of unilateral mesial temporal sclerosis by MRI is valuable information when evaluating a patient for surgery. In one recent review of seven reports in the literature, evaluating a total of 341 patients with epilepsy who had both CT and MRI scans, the MRI was superior in almost all of them. The overall detection rate of abnormalities was 32% for CT and 42% for MRI.[15]

References

1. Hauser WA, Kurland LT: The epidemiology of epilepsy in

Rochester, Minnesota, 1935 through 1967. *Epilepsia* 1975; 16:1-66.

2. Kapoor WN, Karpf M, Wieaned S, et al: A prospective evaluation and follow-up of patients with syncope. *N Engl J Med* 1983;309:197-204.

3. Kerr A Jr, Derbes VJ: The syndrome of cough syncope. *Ann Intern Med* 1953;39:1240-1253.

4. DeMaria AA, Westmoreland BF, Sharbrough FW: EEG in cough syncope. *Neurology* 1984;34:371-374.

5. Peretz DI, Abdulla A: Management of cardioinhibitory hypersensitive carotid sinus syndrome with permanent cardiac pacing: a 17-year prospective study. *Can J Cardiol* 1985; 1:86-91.

6. Schwartz PJ, Periti M, Malliani A: Long QT syndrome. *Am Heart J* 1975;89: 378-390.

7. Ramani SV, Quesney LF, Olson D: Diagnosis of hysterical seizures in epileptic patients. *Am J Psychiatry* 1980; 137:705-709.

8. Lombrosco CT, Lerman P: Breath-holding spells (cyanotic and pallid infantile syncope). *Pediatrics* 1967;39:563-581.

9. Temkin O: *The Falling Sickness: A History of Epilepsy from the Greeks to the Beginnings of Modern Neurology*. 2nd ed, revised. Baltimore and London, Johns Hopkins Press, 1971, p 166.

10. Temkin O: *The Falling Sickness: A History of Epilepsy from the Greeks to the Beginnings of Modern Neurology*. 2nd ed, revised. Baltimore and London, Johns Hopkins Press, 1971, p 327.

11. Berg BO: Neurocutaneous syndromes: phakomatoses and allied conditions. In: *Pediatric Neurology*. Vol 2. Swaiman KF, ed. St Louis, CV Mosby Co, 1989, pp 795-817.

12. Trimble MR: Serum prolactin in epilepsy and hysteria. *Br Med J* 1978;2:1682.

13. Aminoff MJ: Electroencephalography: General principles and clinical applications. In: Aminoff MJ, ed. *Electrodiagnosis in Clinical Neurology*. 2nd ed. New York, Churchill Livingstone, 1986, pp 21-77.

14. White JC, Langston JW, Pedley TA: Benign epileptiform transients of sleep. *Neurology* 1977;27:1061.

15. Riela AR, Penry JK: Magnetic resonance imaging. In: *Comprehensive Epileptology*. Dam M, Gram L, eds. New York, Raven Press, 1990, p 359.

Chapter 5

When to Start and When to Stop Treatment for Seizures

One of the most difficult decisions facing a physician caring for a patient with a seizure is deciding when to start treatment. This decision can be made only after the patient and his or her physician discuss and evaluate a number of issues. The first step is to assess the risk of further seizures.

If the seizures are nonepileptic, treatment must be directed at the underlying cause. Thus, hypoglycemic seizures of the neonate are treated with glucose, alcohol withdrawal seizures can best be controlled by altering addictive behavior, and seizures of psychogenic origin can be modified by appropriate counseling. Treatment of epileptic seizures is governed by assessing the risk of treatment against the benefit of using medications. One of the major reasons for being familiar with epilepsy syndromes is that knowledge of their natural history permits better identification of the risk of further seizures. For example, children with benign epilepsy with centrotemporal spikes may not need treatment with medications because studies have shown that they often outgrow this condition after experiencing only a few nocturnal seizures. Therefore, the overall risk of medication treatment may not be warranted.

Some structural lesions are clearly associated with recurrent seizures. These include brain tumor and arteriovenous malformation. When these are diagnosed after a single seizure, there should be no hesitation in initiating pharmacologic treatment. However, a much more common situation is the one in which the initial evaluation fails to reveal a specific provoking factor (eg, drug abuser, structural lesion, etc). Then the clinician must carefully evaluate the risk of subsequent seizures.

New data from clinical studies in the last decade have identified specific risk factors, based on a complete evaluation, that help identify patients who are at higher risk for having additional seizures.

Table 1
When to Use Chronic Treatment With Antiepileptic Medication After a Single Seizure

If a single seizure is followed rapidly by a second seizure—for example, within the first day—treatment should be started regardless of etiology. An MRI, EEG, and careful examination are needed to make these decisions.

Definitely:

With structural lesion:

- Brain tumor, such as meningioma, glioma, neoplastic
- Arteriovenous malformation
- Infection, such as abscess, herpes encephalitis

Without structural lesion:

- History of epilepsy in sibling (but not parents)
- EEG with definite epileptic pattern
- History of prior acute seizure—a seizure in the context of an illness or a childhood febrile seizure
- History of brain injury or stroke, CNS infection, significant head trauma
- Todd's postictal paresis
- Status epilepticus at onset

Possibly:

- Unprovoked seizure with none of the above risk factors

Probably Not (although short-term therapy may be used):

- Alcohol withdrawal
- Drug abuse
- Seizure in context of acute illness, ie, high fever, dehydration, hypoglycemia
- Postimpact seizure (a single seizure immediately after an acute blow to the head)
- A specific benign epilepsy syndrome such as febrile convulsions or benign epilepsy with centrotemporal spikes
- Seizure provoked by excessive sleep deprivation (eg, college student at examination time)

Categories for Treatment

The decision to treat can be divided into three general categories: treat; possibly treat; and probably not treat, summarized in Table 1. The clinical research supporting these decisions has been developed in a series of papers for adults[1-7] and for children.[8-10]

Studies have found a recurrence rate of 34% to 71% after a single seizure in adults.[1,2] Variance among these studies can be explained in part by differences in study design, characteristics of

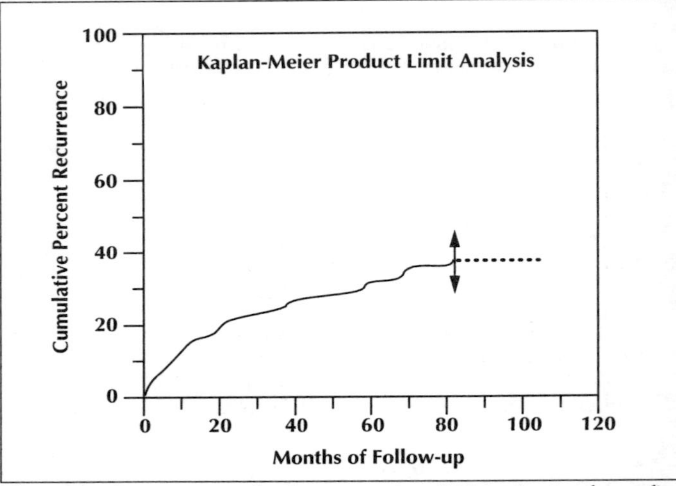

***Figure 1**—Recurrence of seizures among 208 patients after a first unprovoked seizure. Arrows identify standard errors. Used with permission,* Neurology *1990.*[1]

populations, and duration of follow-up. Generally, the longer the follow-up, the higher the rate of recurrence.

A study of 208 patients, all of whom had one unprovoked seizure and were followed for more than 4 years (total of 853 patient years), found an overall risk of 34% for a second seizure at the end of 5 years[1] (Figure 1). Patients for this study (teenagers and adults) were drawn from hospital admissions and referrals to EEG laboratories and neurology and epilepsy clinics at four hospitals (one university hospital, one Veterans Administration hospital, and two urban hospitals).

In this study, patients who had no history of a central nervous system (CNS) insult (idiopathic single seizure) had a recurrence risk of 10% at 1 year, 24% at 2 years, and 29% at 5 years. This group was evaluated for further risk factors. Family history was important. Among those with an idiopathic single seizure and a sibling with seizures, the recurrence rate was 29% at 1 year and 46% at 5 years, compared to 9% at 1 year and 26% at 5 years for those with no sibling with epilepsy (Figure 2).

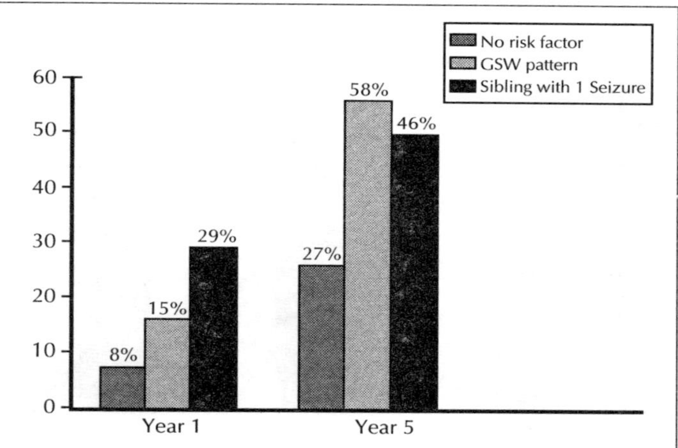

***Figure 2**—The probability of a second seizure 1 and 5 years after a single seizure, based on three sets of factors: no known risk, a generalized spike-wave (GSW) pattern on the EEG, and a sibling with one or more seizures.*[1]

Additionally, a history of seizures in parents or in first-degree relatives was not associated with a higher risk than those patients with idiopathic single seizure.

Another important predictive factor was the EEG. Patients with a pattern of generalized spikes and waves (GSW) had a recurrence risk of 15% at 1 year and 58% at 5 years, compared to 9% and 26%, respectively, for those with normal EEG or nonspecific EEG pattern (Figure 2).

Another important factor was the occurrence of a previous seizure in the context of an illness, or a childhood febrile seizure. These patients had a risk of 10% at 1 year and 39% at 5 years.

Age, gender, seizure type, abnormal EEG other than GSW, and abnormal neurologic examination did not elevate the risk above others in the idiopathic group.

Another group was categorized as "remote symptomatic." These were patients who had a history of head trauma, stroke, CNS infection, or static encephalopathy from birth with mental retardation or cerebral palsy. These patients had a risk for a second seizure of 26% at 1 year, 41% at 2 years, and 48% at 5 years, markedly higher than idiopathic rates of 10%, 24%, and

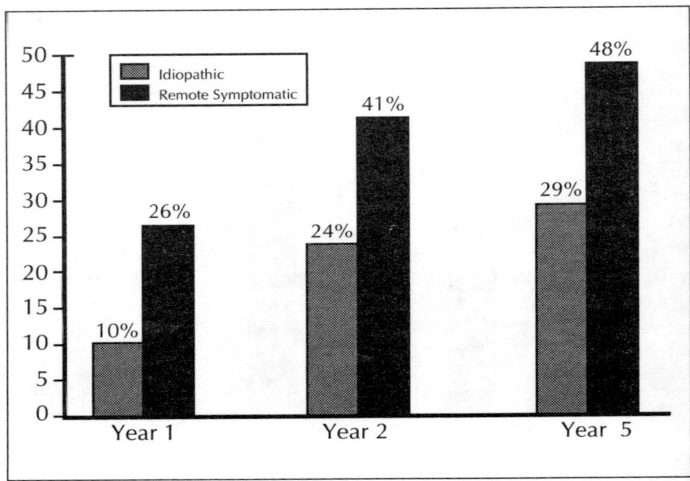

***Figure 3**—Recurrence risk for idiopathic (no known central nervous system injury) or remote symptomatic (previous stroke, head injury, infection, etc).*[1]

29%, respectively (Figure 3).

Within the remote symptomatic group, increased risk for recurrence was found in those with Todd's postictal paresis—41% at 1 year and 75% at 5 years. If a prior acute seizure was present, the risk for a second seizure was 60% at 1 year and 80% at 5 years. If status epilepticus or multiple seizures occurred at onset, the recurrence rate was 37% at 1 year and 56% at 3 years.

Thus, a patient with a previous CNS insult, or with a sibling with seizures, or with prior acute seizure, or with a GSW-EEG pattern, or with Todd's postictal paresis, has a significantly higher risk of a second seizure than a patient without these risk factors. Most neurologists would treat these patients with antiepileptic medications.

When Risk Factors Are Lacking

A more difficult decision arises for those patients with none of the additional risk factors. For these patients, the probability of a second seizure is less than 10% in the first year and approximately 24% by the end of 2 years after the single seizure. Is this a high enough rate to warrant the risks of treatment? There is no single answer to this question. The decision to treat or not to treat must be based on an evaluation by the patient and physician of the perceived risk and benefit. As described in other sections, the risk of treatment with available antiepileptic medications is generally low. The impact of a second seizure depends on the patient's life-style. Treatment may be indicated for patients needing to drive, or for those who face significant risk of injury or loss of self-esteem from a second seizure. The risk of recurrence is greatest in the first 2 years, so if treatment is initiated, it probably can be halted after the highest risk period passes.

Treatment is predicated on the assumption that recurrent seizures can be prevented with adequate medication. In the Hauser study,[1] treatment with antiepileptic medication was initially recommended for 80% of all cases. There did not appear to be a difference in recurrence rates between treated and untreated patients. This lack of effect may be explained by the study design, which was an observational and not an interventional analysis. Thus, compliance, uniformity of treatment, and other variables were not controlled. Only a few studies have examined treatment after a single seizure. One study randomized half of 397 patients aged 2 to 70 years to treatment with an antiepileptic drug after a single unprovoked generalized tonic-clonic seizure. The treated group had a calculated risk of seizure recurrence of 25% at 24 months, compared to 51% for the untreated persons.[11] Thus, limited clinical studies and intuition would suggest that treatment may prevent some but not all persons from having additional seizures.

In considering the issue of when to treat, social as well as therapeutic factors must be taken into account. For an adult, the most important question is that of driving a motor vehicle. In most cases, a single seizure has not been considered grounds for restricting driving, but the presence of epilepsy as demonstrated by the occurrence of two or more seizures subjects the patient to numerous restrictions. Thus, some patients, after reviewing the odds with their physician, elect to begin treatment after a single seizure. These decisions are difficult and should never be made unilaterally by the physician for the patient. Rather, the patient should be aware of the risks and benefits of the alternative strategies, and the key elements of the decision must be recorded in the medical record. In children, there may be less pressure to treat and the side effect profile may be less beneficial than in adults.[9,10] Also, identification of a specific epilepsy syndrome in a child can be useful in deciding whether to treat.

As shown in Figure 1, the steepest part of the recurrence rate curve is in the first 24 months, when the possibility of a second seizure is highest. Some physicians prefer to treat for 2 years in the case when the patient has no major risk factors but wishes to have protection from recurrence.

When to Stop Treatment

The decision to stop treatment must be made with the same consideration of the probability of recurrent seizures as in the decision to start treatment. Many older textbooks advised that treatment could be stopped after 2 years of seizure control. But this recommendation is not valid in the context of present knowledge of epileptic syndromes. As discussed briefly in Chapter 3, some epileptic syndromes are age-specific, and some patients mature to the stage of low risk. For example, children with benign epilepsy with centrotemporal spikes "outgrow" their seizures regardless of treatment. For other syndromes, however, there is a lifelong tendency for seizures to occur, and control of such seizures is not an indication that the disorder is in remission. A person with an arteriovenous malformation may achieve complete control for many years but remain at risk for seizures if medication is discontinued.

In one recent study, patients (mostly adults) who had been seizure-free for at least 4 years were asked to participate in a study of withdrawal of medication. Of 62 who elected to enter the withdrawal phase, 15 (24%) had a recurrent seizure. Of the 157 who declined to withdraw from medication, 10 (6%) had a seizure.[12] In another study evaluating 1,013 patients who were seizure-free for at least 2 years, patients were prospectively randomized to withdrawal or continuation of treatment. In the continuing treatment group, 12% had subsequent seizures, while in the slow withdrawal group 41% had subsequent seizures.[13] The factors that appeared to be related to successful withdrawal were: single type of seizure; normal neurologic examination; normal IQ; and normal EEG following treatment. Thus, benefits of withdrawal (freedom from daily medication, reduction of side effects, decreased risk of teratogenic effects [Chapter 10]) must be balanced against a 20% to 30% probability of seizure recurrence (loss of job, possible injury). Whatever the decision, it must be made with the patient's full understanding of the risks involved. Medication should never be stopped abruptly because this may lead to withdrawal seizures or to status epilepticus. Rather, medications should be tapered over months, depending on the nature of the medication. Phenobarbital, with a long half-life and great potential for causing withdrawal seizures, should be withdrawn over many months, usually in increments of 25% of the initial dose. Phenytoin, carbamazepine, and valproate may be withdrawn over 6 to 10 weeks.

References

1. Hauser WA, Rich SS, et al: Seizure recurrence after a first unprovoked seizure: an extended follow-up. *Neurology* 1990; 40:1163-1170.

2. Ewles RDC, Reynolds EH: Should people be treated after a first seizure? *Arch Neurol* 1988; 45:490-491.

3. Annegers JF, Grabow JD, Groover RV, et al: Seizures after head trauma: a population study. *Neurology* 1980;30:683-689.

4. Annegers JF, Shirts SB, Hauser WA, et al: Risk of recurrence after an initial unprovoked seizure. *Epilepsia* 1986; 27:43-50.

5. Hart RG, Easton JD: Seizure recurrence after a first, unprovoked seizure. *Arch Neurol* 1988;43: 1289-1290.

6. Hauser WA, Ramiraz-Lassepas M, Rosenstein R: Risk for seizures and epilepsy following cerebrovascular insults. *Epilepsia* 1984;25:666. Abstract.

7. Hopkins A, Garman A, Clarke C: The first seizure in adult life. *Lancet* 1988;1:721-726.

8. Benedetti MD, Shinnar S, Cohen H, et al: Risk factors for epilepsy in children with cerebral palsy and/or mental retardation. *Epilepsia* 1986;27:614. Abstract.

9. Camfield PR, Camfield CS, Dooley JM, et al: Epilepsy after a first unprovoked seizure in childhood. *Neurology* 1985;35: 1657-1660.

10. Shinnar S, Berg D, Moshe SL, et al: The risk of seizure recurrence following a first unprovoked seizure in childhood: a prospective study. *Pediatrics* 1990;85:1076-1085.

11. First Seizure Trial Group. Randomized clinical trial on the efficacy of antiepileptic drugs in reducing the risk of relapse after a first unprovoked tonic-clonic seizure. *Neurology* 1993;43:478-483.

12. Dean JC, Penry PK: Remission and relapse in chronic epilepsy. *Epilepsia* 1990;31(5):648. Abstract.

13. Chadwick D: Randomized study of AED withdrawal in patients in remission. Medical Research Council, AED Withdrawal Study Group. *Lancet* 1991;337: 1175-1180.

Chapter 6

Principles of Treatment

The goal of treatment with antiepileptic drugs (AEDs) is to prevent the recurrence of seizures while avoiding side effects from the drugs. Treatment of epilepsy requires that both the physician and the patient understand the goals and time frame of treatment. Because no one can predict precisely when another seizure will occur, AEDs must be used so that therapeutic concentrations of the drug, its metabolites, or its biochemical effector are present in the central nervous system for the period of risk. Moreover, because patients can have long intervals between seizures with no intervening symptoms, the issue of compliance becomes critical. The most common cause of treatment failure is noncompliance.[1]

Considerable discussion exists about how to select the best AED to treat a patient's epilepsy. Some large, well-controlled studies provide guidance in helping the clini-

Table 1
Selecting AEDs Based on Classification of Seizures and Epileptic Syndromes

Seizure or Syndrome Type	Effective Drugs
Partial	*First line*
simple, complex, and secondarily generalized	carbamazepine phenytoin valproate gabapentin lamotrigine vigabatrin
	Second line
	phenobarbital primidone felbamate
Generalized	
absence	ethosuximide valproate
myoclonic	clonazepam valproate
tonic-clonic	valproate carbamazepine phenytoin
Lennox-Gastaut	valproate felbamate clonazepam phenobarbital

cian and patient make an effective choice. Accurately identifying the seizure type and the epileptic syndrome is very helpful in choosing the drug for the best outcome (Table 1). Localization-related epilepsies usually respond well to carbamazepine, felbamate, gabapentin, lamotrigine, phenytoin, phenobarbital, primidone, and valproate. Studies have shown that carbamazepine and phenytoin are likely to be successful as initial treatment in adults.[2-5] The role of the newer drugs as initial treatment is being evaluated. Generalized epilepsies usually respond best to valproate and the benzodiazepines. Ethosuximide is effective for absence seizures but not for partial seizures; so in a patient with brief spells, the differential between these must be carefully made. Myoclonic seizures respond well to clonazepam and valproate. Persons with juvenile myoclonic epilepsy (JME) often respond well to valproate, but not to carbamazepine or phenytoin. Thus, if a young person presents with a generalized tonic-clonic seizure, the clinician must differentiate between a localization-related epilepsy and JME.

In adults, the most common seizure type is a partial seizure with secondary generalized, that is, localization-related epilepsy. One early study comparing phenytoin and carbamazepine as initial therapy evaluated 70 patients who were followed for 6 months to 2 years.[2] Treatment failure (defined as continued occurrence of seizures despite doses of medications that produced toxic symptoms) occurred in 5 of 35 patients receiving carbamazepine, and in 4 of 35 patients receiving phenytoin. Of the patients without major side effects in whom efficacy of a single medication could be evaluated, control was obtained in 81.5% of the carbamazepine-treated group (22 of 27 patients) and in 85.8% of the phenytoin-treated group (23 of 27 patients).

The mean dosage of carbamazepine ranged from 3.38 to 16.48 mg/kg/day (mean 9.32 ± 3.16 mg/kg/day), and that of phenytoin ranged from 2.2 to 9.9 mg/kg/day (mean 5.35 ± 1.74 mg/kg/day). Mean serum blood levels associated with successful therapy in weeks 8 through 24 were 9.1 to 11.0 mg/L with phenytoin, and 4.7 to 6.5 mg/L with carbamazepine.

The largest study to date (622 patients) of treatment efficacy was a multicenter Veterans Administration hospital (VAH) study that compared carbamazepine, phenytoin, primidone, and phenobarbital.[3] Patients were randomized to one of these four drugs, but were switched to another if toxicity occurred or if seizures were not controlled. Overall, the total seizure control was only 39% at 12 months and was similar with all the drugs tested (carbamazepine 47%, phenytoin 38%, phenobarbital 36%, and primidone 35%). The prognosis for complete control of tonic-clonic seizures with the four drugs was also similar (carbamazepine 48%, phenytoin 43%, phenobarbital 43%, and primidone, 45%). Partial seizures were controlled with phenobarbital in 16%, with primidone in 15%, with phenytoin in 26%, and with carbamazepine in 43%. The difference in control between carbamazepine and phenytoin was not statistically significant but carbamazepine was statistically superior to phenobarbital and primidone.[3] Overall, for seizure control and toxicity, phenytoin and carbamazepine were similar, and both were superior to phenobarbital and primidone (Figure 1).

One review of 20 trials evaluated 1,336 adult patients with newly diagnosed, presumed localization-related epilepsy. All

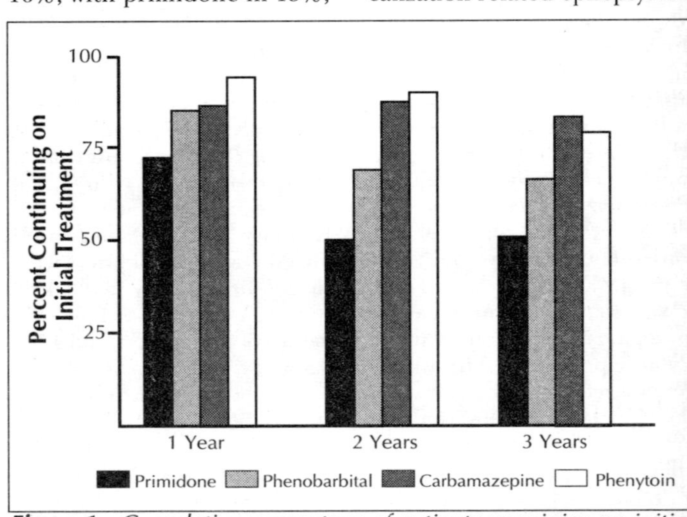

***Figure 1**—Cumulative percentage of patients remaining on initial drug (successfully treated) with primidone, phenobarbital, carbamazepine, and phenytoin, during 36 months of follow-up.*
(Adapted from information appearing in The New England Journal of Medicine.*)*[3]

the trials met the criterion of incorporating a prospective, randomized, double-blind design. But no significant difference was found in efficacy among the medications tested.[4] Thus, no well-controlled study has shown a significant difference in efficacy between carbamazepine and phenytoin, and choices must be made on factors other than efficacy alone.

Valproate has also been evaluated as treatment for complex-partial seizures. A recent VAH cooperative study found it to be slightly less effective than carbamazepine.[5] Another study, however, found no difference between phenytoin, valproate, and carbamazepine.[6]

Studies comparing the safety of AEDs have shown that different drugs have different side effect profiles. Perhaps the most detailed of these comparisons was the VAH cooperative study.[3] In that study, many of the patients who withdrew from the study did so because of untoward side effects associated with primidone and phenobarbital. Thus, while all four drugs had similar efficacy, the cumulative percentage of patients retained in the study for 36 months was the lowest for primidone and phenobarbital because of toxicity-associated failure (Figure 1).

Various systemic and neurotoxic effects occurred with all four drugs, but some were significantly more common or less common with specific drugs.[3] Phenobarbital was associated with the lowest incidence of motor disturbance (ataxia, uncoordination, nystagmus, and tremor) early in treatment. Phenytoin caused more dysmorphic and idiosyncratic side effects—including gum hypertrophy, hirsutism, acne, and rash—than other drugs (carbamazepine 14%; phenobarbital 11%; phenytoin 22%; and primidone 10%). Reports of decreased libido or impotence were most frequent among patients given primidone.

Potentially life-threatening side effects were very infrequent. Successful treatment considered both efficacy and side effects. Figure 1 depicts the cumulative percentage of patients successfully treated with each drug during a 36-month follow-up period.

Treatment should be started with a single drug. Some years ago, it was popular to initiate treatment with both phenobarbital and phenytoin, based on the belief that these drugs had a synergistic action. However, the effect of these drugs in the central nervous system was shown to be additive and

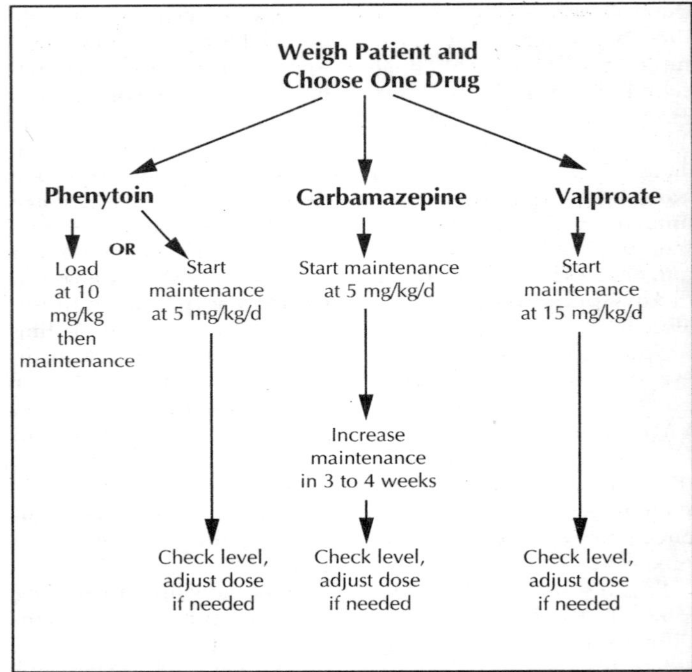

Figure 2*—Initiation of treatment with antiepileptic medication in adults. Doses may be larger for children or smaller for the elderly.*

there is no longer a rationale for initiating treatment with more than one medication.[7] Studies have shown that up to 80% of patients with new onset epilepsy can be successfully controlled with one medication.[8] However, if the first drug is not effective, another drug useful for the same category of seizures should be started. Some patients with intractable epilepsy will need more than one drug to control seizures.

Initiation of treatment can be done either by starting a maintenance dose or by using a loading dose followed by a maintenance dose (Figure 2). Most often, the treatment is started by using the maintenance dose. However, because

Table 2
Titration of Phenytoin

To attain the appropriate concentrations, use 100-mg and 30-mg doses of phenytoin to titrate in small increments. Dose increments of 10 mg are possible. Because there is a difference in mg of phenytoin between the capsule (sodium salt) and Infatabs®, titration with capsules rather than the 50-mg Infatabs is recommended. Some examples of combinations are:

Total daily dose	Number of 100 mg	Number of 30 mg
200	2	
230	2	1
260	2	2
290	2	3
300	3	0
310	1	7
320	2	4
330	3	1
360	3	2
400	4	

five half-lives are needed to reach a steady-state level, loading is preferred in some instances. Knowledge of pharmacokinetic principles can be useful in developing initiation and maintenance strategies.

Initiation With Phenytoin

Because of its pK_a, phenytoin is not absorbed in the stomach, but must pass into the small intestine where the pH becomes alkaline. Thus, phenytoin absorption begins a few hours after administration and reaches its peak 6 to 12 hours later. Despite its slow absorption, the bioavailability of phenytoin is good; about 90% of an oral dose is absorbed. There is a difference in presently available products. Dilantin® has a slower absorption rate than generic formulations and there is no allowable substitution at this time.

Maintenance treatment with phenytoin in the adult can be started with 5 mg/kg/day. For many adults, this will be approximately 300 mg. Dosage adjustments should be made to meet individual requirements.

If phenytoin is started as maintenance, it will take 5 to 7 days to reach steady-state concentration (five half-lives). But this may not be acceptable, especially if the patient is expected to be discharged from the hospital shortly, or if the patient has an acute series of seizures. In these cases, loading doses may be used. This dosing regimen should be used in a clinic or hospital where phenytoin serum levels can be monitored closely.

Intravenous phenytoin has a volume of distribution (V_d) of 0.78 L/kg. Thus, an IV dose of 0.78 mg/kg will increase the blood level by 1.0 mg/L. Clinicians can tailor the dose to attain any specific desired blood level. For example, if one wishes to increase the blood level by 10 mg/L, one needs to give a dose of 7.8 mg/kg. For a 60-kg patient, this is approximately 480 mg.

For oral loading, it is more difficult to calculate a precise volume of distribution because absorption is competing with metabolism. Studies have shown that doses of approximately 1 mg/kg will raise the blood levels by 1 mg/kg. Partial loading may be useful if an increase in levels is needed. For example, suppose a patient who has been well controlled by phenytoin concentrations of 15 mg/L has a breakthrough seizure. The patient is taken to the emergency department, where a concentration of 5 mg/L is recorded. Then the physician can give a dose of 10 mg/kg to restore the level to 15.

During steady state, the dose must be sufficient to maintain the desired blood concentration. For an average adult, doses of 4 to 6 mg/kg per day are sufficient to maintain blood levels in the therapeutic range. For this reason, the patient's weight must be known. A standard dose of 300 mg/day may be sufficient for patients in the 60-kg range, but will be too high for patients weighing only 40 kg. On the other hand, patients weighing more than 100 kg (220 lbs) will be underdosed if given 300 mg/day and instead need 500 mg/day.

Children are more rapid metabolizers of phenytoin than are adults. Children may need doses two or three times greater than adults on a mg-per-kg basis (8 to 10 mg/kg). Thus, a child weighing 30 kg may need 300 mg/day of phenytoin. The 30-mg capsules are useful for adjusting doses precisely (Table 2).

As patients grow older, there is a reduction in the cytochrome P-450 system, and doses used for adults may be too high for the elderly. Consequently, doses of 3 to 4 mg/kg/day may be more appropriate for the elderly. However, we lack good studies regarding dosing in this age group.

Another issue is protein

binding. Phenytoin is approximately 90% protein bound, and the usual methods for measuring this drug yield total concentrations, that is, both bound and unbound (free). The elderly may have lower albumin levels, so the total concentrations for them may be lower than for comparable "free" levels. For example, a patient with normal binding with a concentration of 15 mg/L would have a "free" level of 1.5 mg/L, and a bound level of 13.5 mg/L. However, if the binding is affected by low albumin, the unbound fraction may be 20% of the total, or 3.0 mg/L. This would be the equivalent of a total level of 30 mg/L in a patient with normal binding. Thus, if an elderly person exhibits symptoms of toxicity, but his or her total levels of phenytoin are in the therapeutic range, an unbound concentration should be obtained, or, more simply, the dose should be reduced to attain a lower steady-state level. In the elderly, total phenytoin concentrations of 5 to 10 mg/L may be sufficient. Another problem arises from drug interactions that can displace phenytoin from binding sites.

Initiation With Carbamazepine

Carbamazepine dosage must be adjusted for each patient. Because it has a long half-life on initiation of therapy, doses of 200 mg b.i.d. are recommended for adults. Doses may be increased at weekly intervals by adding up to 200 mg/day using a t.i.d. or q.i.d. regimen until the best response is obtained. Doses should not generally exceed 1g/day in children 12 to 15 years of age, and should not exceed 1.2 g/day in patients 16 years of age or older. However, doses up to 2 g/day have been used in adults in some cases. Children 6 to 11 years of age should have an initial dose of 100 mg b.i.d., and doses can be increased at weekly intervals using a t.i.d. or q.i.d. regimen until the best response is obtained. Generally, doses of 5 to 8 mg/kg/day are sufficient during the first week of treatment but may need to be increased to 10 to 15 mg/kg/day with chronic use.

The half-life becomes shorter with chronic use because of autoinduction of carbamazepine metabolism, so the dosing interval may need to be increased to t.i.d. or q.i.d. Protein binding of carbamazepine is usually not clinically important. The major metabolite of carbamazepine, the 10,11 epoxide, also has antiepileptic properties and toxicity. Standard methods for measuring carbamazepine do not measure its epoxide. Usually, the epoxide is less than 20% of the parent drug, and at low levels causes no problems. However, some patients are deficient in epoxide hydrolase and valproate inhibits this enzyme that metabolizes this compound. Patients may exhibit toxicity with a carbamazepine concentration lower than one usually associates with symptoms. Most laboratories will be able to send samples to regional reference laboratories for epoxide determinations.

Carbamazepine use in the elderly has not been well studied. In general, doses may need to be lower on a mg/kg/day basis. Also, carbamazepine may interact with some medications used in the elderly.

Initiation With Valproate

The recommended initial dose of valproate is 15 mg/kg/day. Since valproate does not induce its own metabolism, doses do not need to be increased unless the patient is not obtaining full control. Doses may be increased at 1-week intervals by 5 to 10 mg/kg/day until seizures are controlled or until side effects preclude further increases. The maximum recommended dose is 60 mg/kg/day. Valproate is not widely used in the elderly and there are little data regarding its use in this group.

Monitoring Treatment

After AED therapy is initiated, treatment should be monitored for two important reasons: to evaluate the effectiveness of the AED, and to determine the drug's safety. Evaluating the effectiveness of treatment is best done by recording the patient's seizures accurately. It is recommended that patients with epilepsy record their seizures on a calendar so that an accurate assessment of effectiveness can be made. When a patient is doing well, with no seizures and no side effects, a blood level should be obtained to have a benchmark, or target, for that individual. This can be used in the future to determine control. If a patient has a breakthrough seizure and the level is significantly lower than the benchmark, noncompliance can be suspected. Then the physician can institute education and other means to foster compliance. If the level is at the benchmark, the target level can then be raised, on the conclusion that the seizure threshold is higher.

AEDs have been associated with rare, fatal aplastic anemia

and hepatic failure. For this reason, it is necessary to obtain baseline values of hepatic and hematopoietic parameters. Some clinicians monitor these parameters every 3 to 6 months. Some studies, however, indicate that the most cost-effective monitoring is done when patients are experiencing symptoms (Chapter 10).

It is useful to measure AED levels annually to assure that compliance is being maintained and to confirm that there have been no significant changes in metabolism of the drugs. This is particularly important if the physician is taking responsibility for certifying eligibility for the patient's driving privileges.

References

1. Leppik IE, Schmidt D: Summary of the First International Workshop on Compliance in Epilepsy. *Epilepsy Res* 1988;1(suppl):179-182.

2. Ramsay RE, Wilder BJ, Berger JR, et al: A double-blind study comparing carbamazepine with phenytoin as initial seizure therapy in adults. *Neurology* 1975;33:904-910.

3. Mattson RH, Cramer JA, Collins JF, et al: Comparison of carbamazepine, phenobarbital, phenytoin, and primidone in partial and secondarily generalized tonic-clonic seizures. *N Engl J Med* 1985; 313:145-151.

4. Treiman DM: Efficacy and safety of antiepileptic drugs: a review of controlled trials. *Epilepsia* 1987;28(suppl 3):S1-S8.

5. Mattson RH, et al: Valproate vs carbamazepine for seizures, a comparison of valproate with carbamazepine for the treatment of complex partial seizures and secondarily generalized tonic-clonic seizures in adults. *N Engl J Med* 1992;327(11):765.

6. Callaghan N, Kenny RA, O'Neill B, et al: A prospective study between carbamazepine, phenytoin, and sodium valproate as monotherapy in previously untreated and recently diagnosed patients with epilepsy. *J Neurol Neurosurg Psychiatry* 1985;48:639-644.

7. Leppik IE, Sherwin AL: Anticonvulsant activity of phenobarbital and phenytoin in combination. *J Pharmacol Exp Ther* 1977;200:570-576.

8. Reynolds EH, Chadwick D, Galbraith AW: One drug (phenytoin) in the treatment of epilepsy. *Lancet* 1976;1:923-926.

Chapter 7

Standard Antiepileptic Drugs (AEDs)

This chapter examines in detail information about the specific attributes of the standard antiepileptic drugs (AEDs). It summarizes each drug's actions and uses, pharmacokinetics, doses and preparations, adverse reactions, and common drug interactions. Table 1 is a summary of the doses and levels of the standard AEDs.

History of Antiepileptic Medications

The first effective drug for treatment of epileptic seizures was bromide. In 1857, Locock, in a discussion of a paper on the

Table 1
Doses and Plasma Concentrations of Standard Antiepileptic Drugs

Drug	Average Daily Maintenance Dose: Adults (mg)	Adults (mg/kg)	Children (mg/kg)	Usually Effective Plasma Concentrations (mg/L)*
Carbamazepine	600 mg–1.2 g	5–15	15–30	4–12
Phenytoin	300–400 mg	4–6	6–8	10–20
Valproate	750 mg–1.0 g (monotherapy)	15–25 (monotherapy)	15–20 (monotherapy)	40–120
	1.5–3.0 g (combination therapy)	30–60 (combination therapy)	30–100 (combination therapy)	
Clonazepam	2–6 mg	0.1–0.2	0.1–0.2	0.02–0.08
Ethosuximide	500 mg–2.0 g	15–40	15–40	40–100
Phenobarbital	120–250 mg	2–3	3–5	15–40
Primidone	750 mg–1.5 g	8–16	10–25	5–12

*Concentrations are reported as µg/mL by some laboratories, but mg/L is the preferred unit and will be used in this book. 1 µg/mL= 1 mg/L

etiology of seizures, disclosed that he had had remarkable success using bromide in female patients with intractable epilepsy. His experience was confirmed by others, and soon tons of bromide were being used as primary therapy for epilepsy.

Table 2
Antiepileptic Drugs Marketed in the United States

Year Introduced	Name
1912	phenobarbital
1935	mephobarbital
1938	phenytoin
1947	mephenytoin
1949	paramethadione
1951	phenacemide
1953	phensuximide
1954	primidone
1957	methsuximide
1957	ethotoin
1960	ethosuximide
1968	diazepam
1974	carbamazepine
1975	clonazepam
1978	valproate
1981	clorazepate
1993	felbamate
	gabapentin
1994	lamotrigine
1996	vigabatrin
	Withdrawn Drugs
1946	trimethadione
1950	phenthenylate
1952	metharbital
1952	benzchlorpropamide
1960	aminoglutethimide

Before the introduction of bromide, almost every conceivable potion, diet, and ritual had been used without significant benefit. Although effective for controlling seizures, bromide's side effects are considerable and include sedation, depression, skin eruptions, and gastrointestinal distress. For more than 60 years, bromide was the only effective substance known for the treatment of epilepsy. Because sedation was a prominent side effect of bromide, it was considered by many to be essential for anticonvulsant effect. Based on this concept, Hauptmann proposed using phenobarbital for the treatment of epilepsy in 1912. For the next 25 years, epilepsy was treated with drugs associated with slowing of mentation, and in retrospect, much of the belief that persons with epilepsy were mentally subnormal may have been a result of the treatment rather than the disorder.

Today, it is difficult to imagine that substances to treat illnesses could be given to humans before being thoroughly tested in animals for safety and efficacy, but this had been the case for millennia. It was only in the early part of this century that the scientific community and the public began to see the value of animal testing prior to exposure in humans.[1]

Table 3: Pharmacokinetic Data on Standard Antiepileptic Drugs*

Drug	Time to Steady State (Days)	Plasma Half-Life (Hours)			
		Adults		Children	
		Mean	Range	Mean	Range
Carbamazepine	21–28	10–20[a]	5–26	8–14	3–25
Clonazepam	6		18–50		22–33
Ethosuximide	7–10	52–56	40–60	30–36	15–68
Phenobarbital	>21	96	53–140	67–72	37–133
Phenytoin	6–8[b]	20–30[c]	8–59		
Primidone	4–7	15	4–22 (mono-therapy)	10	(mono-therapy
		9	3–11 (poly-therapy)	8	(poly-therapy
Valproate	1–4		12–16 (mono-therapy)		8–12 (mono-therapy
		8	5–10 (polytherapy)	8	5–9 (polythera

[a] *Initially the average half-life is 30 to 35 hours; values listed are after autoinduction.*

[b] *May be 2 to 3 weeks if plasma concentrations are above 20 mg/L.*

*Modified from *Drug Evaluations Annual 1991*, used with permission

The work of Merritt and Putnam with phenytoin demonstrated that the use of an animal model of seizures was an efficient way to screen a large number of compounds for antiepileptic effectiveness. Their work also showed that sedation and depression were not essential for anticonvulsant effect.[2] The subsequent introduction of antiepileptic drugs was rapid. Trimethadione was introduced in 1946, and to 1978, 16 other

Volume [of Di]stribution (L/kg)	Plasma Protein Binding (%)	Elimination Site
0.8–1.4	75	hepatic
1.5–4.4	85	hepatic
0.67	<5	hepatic
0.5–1.0	40–60	hepatic and renal
0.5–1.0	90	hepatic
0.8	20	hepatic and renal
0.15	80–94[d]	hepatic

[c] *Half-life increases with dose.*
[d] *Percent bound decreases as total plasma concentration increases above 75-100 mg/L.*

substances were approved for marketing in the United States. Of these, five have been subsequently withdrawn (Table 2). Most of the others have been found to have only limited utility and are infrequently used.

From 1961 through 1973, no major new drugs for epilepsy were marketed in the United States, although carbamazepine, valproate, and other agents were being used in other countries. Carbamazepine was approved for marketing in the United States in 1974. Valproate was approved in 1978, and then there were no new major drugs approved for the treatment of epilepsy until 1993. Nevertheless, there were significant advances in the use of antiepileptic drugs. This knowledge was acquired by the emergence of new technology to measure antiepileptic drug concentrations in the blood. Previous dosage schedules that were derived solely from clinical experience were replaced by dosage schedules based on pharmacokinetic principles. Additionally, it became possible to determine patient compliance with prescribed therapy.

Unfortunately, noncompliance is much more common than was previously suspected.[3] Depending on the community, as many as 90% of patients attending epilepsy clinics have been found to have levels of antiepileptic drugs below the therapeutic range. Thus, much of the per-

Table 4
Drug Interactions*

	Other AEDs whose levels are affected by the AED in left column		AED affecting level of AED in left column		Other medications affecting level of AED in left column	
Drug	**Increase**	**Decrease**	**Increase**	**Decrease**	**Increase**	**Decrease**
Carbamazepine		clonazepam ethosuximide primidone valproate phenytoin[1] phenobarbital[1]		phenobarbital[1] phenytoin[1]	erythromycin isoniazid propoxyphene troleandomycin cimetidine danazol diltiazem verapamil	
Phenytoin		carbamazepine[1] phenobarbital[1] primidone[1] valproate[1]		carbamazepine[1] phenobarbital[1] valproate[1]	chloramphenicol cimetidine dicumarol disulfiram isoniazid phenylbutazone sulfonamides trimethoprim amiodarone allopurinol chlorpheniramine trazodone	diazoxide antineoplastics loxapine rifampin

Valproate	phenobarbital carbamazepine[4]	phenytoin[3] ethosuximide[1]		carbamazepine phenobarbital primidone phenytoin	salicylates	
Clonazepam	No consistent change in other antiepileptic plasma concentrations noted			 phenobarbital primidone	carbamazepine disulfiram oral contraceptives	cimetidine
Ethosuximide	phenytoin[2]			carbamazepine phenobarbital phenytoin primidone		
Phenobarbital		phenytoin[1] carbamazepine[1] clonazepam	valproate	carbamazepine phenytoin[1]	chloramphenicol propoxyphene	
Primidone	Same as phenobarbital		Same as phenobarbital		isoniazid	

[1] Variable effects (increase, decrease, no change) reported.

[2] Possibly; clinical importance not established.

[3] Variable effects on free and total plasma concentrations.

[4] Increases the carbamazepine epoxide/carbamazepine ratio.

* Modified from *Drug Evaluations Annual 1991*, used with permission.

Table 5
Biologically Active Compounds in Blood

Drug	Biologically Active Compounds in Blood
Carbamazepine	carbamazepine carbamazepine 10,11 epoxide
Clonazepam	clonazepam
Ethosuximide	ethosuximide
Phenobarbital	phenobarbital
Phenytoin	phenytoin
Primidone	primidone phenobarbital phenylethyl malonamide
Valproate	valproic acid 2-en-valproic acid

ceived lack of effectiveness observed by patients and physicians could be caused by patients' lack of adequate drug compliance.

Another important development was the acceptance of an international classification of epileptic seizures and the epilepsy syndromes (Table 1, Chapter 2, and Table 1, Chapter 3). This made the evaluation of current and new drugs more rational. Also, developments in the knowledge of the mechanism of action and of the biochemical mechanisms underlying the genesis of seizures have opened up new avenues of drug development.

Starting in the late 1970s, a renewed interest occurred in developing new drugs for epilepsy treatment in the United States. The Epilepsy Branch of the National Institutes of Health began a comprehensive system for screening promising compounds in animal models of epilepsy. More than 17,000 compounds have been screened, and from these a few were promising enough to warrant testing in humans. During the past decade, more than 15 compounds have been tested in humans in the United States. Under present FDA regulations that require both efficacy and safety to be demonstrated in scientifically valid clinical trials in hundreds of patients, much effort has been expended to develop new drugs or new formulations of presently marketed compounds. It is likely that during the 1990s, touted as the "decade of the brain," many new compounds and some new formulations will become available. Some of the new AEDs are examined in Chapter 8.

Pharmacokinetic properties influence how drugs should be

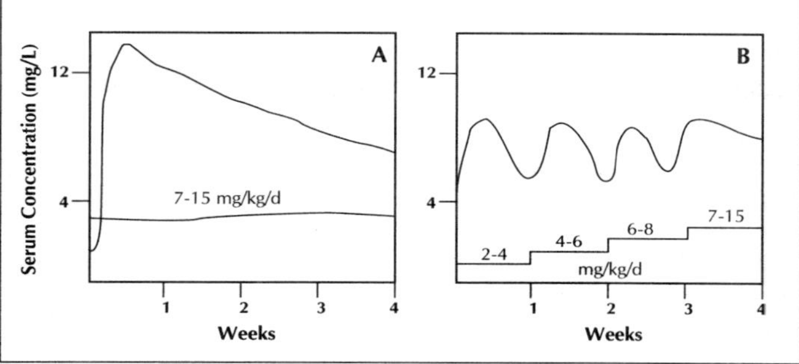

Figure 1*—Hypothetical example of effect of carbamazepine autoinduction. If a large dose is used initially, before induction, toxic levels may result (A). Carbamazepine dose should be increased over the first month of treatment to permit the establishment of stable levels (B).*

dosed; in general, the dose interval should be shorter than the half-life. There is a considerable change in half-life with age: children have the shortest, adults longer, and elderly and newborns the longest (Table 3).

Drug interactions are a major problem. Phenytoin, carbamazepine, and phenobarbital are potent stimulators of hepatic enzyme systems, and can affect concentrations of other AEDs as well as alter concentrations of other prescribed or over-the-counter drugs. This is a particularly important problem in the elderly, many of whom require other medications (Table 4). Drug interactions from AEDs, although somewhat predictable, will vary from patient to patient. Generally, a drug that stimulates hepatic metabolism will lower concentrations of other drugs that use the liver for detoxification. However, by blocking some enzyme systems, drugs can also increase the concentrations by inhibiting metabolism. For highly protein-bound drugs, displacement from binding sites will lower the total serum concentration without necessarily affecting the biological activity. Some AEDs have active metabolites (Table 5).

Carbamazepine: Action and Uses

Carbamazepine (Tegretol®) is effective alone or with other AEDs in partial seizures, especially complex partial seizures, in generalized tonic-clonic seizures, and in combinations of these seizure types. It is ineffective for absence, myoclonic, and atonic seizures. Carbamazepine may exacerbate some generalized seizures with spike-and-wave EEG patterns in children.[4]

Comparative clinical trial data indicate that carbamazepine is better tolerated than phenobarbital and primidone in simple and complex partial seizures, but individual responses vary.[5] This drug is increasingly preferred to phenobarbital in pediatric patients because it appears to have less effect than phenobarbital on cognition and behavior.

Pharmacokinetics

Oral absorption of carbamazepine is variable; peak plasma concentrations occur in 4 to 12 hours after use of solid dosage forms. Bioavailability is estimated at 85%, but may be less when the drug is taken with meals. Rate of absorption may vary with different prescriptions. With monotherapy, the usual effective plasma concentration is 4 to 12 mg/L, but higher concentrations may be required in some patients to control seizures. With concomitant use of other AEDs, low concentrations may be associated with toxicity.

Carbamazepine is metabolized in the liver to its 10,11-epoxide. This compound has both anticonvulsant and toxic effects.[6] Carbamazepine induces its own metabolism; as a result, the usual initial half-life (18 to 35 hours) is reduced considerably after 3 or 4 weeks of administration (Figure 1). Children metabolize carbamazepine faster than adults do and they need larger doses (Table 1). Because of autoinduction of metabolism, plasma concentrations should be monitored during the first month of treatment. Also, because concomitant use of phenytoin or phenobarbital may further induce this metabolic pathway, significantly larger doses of carbamazepine often are required when it is used in combination with these other antiepileptic drugs.

Dosage and Preparations

Oral: Children 6 to 12 years, 100 mg twice daily on the first day. The amount can be increased by 100 mg daily at appropriate intervals (usually 1 to 2 weeks) and given in three or four divided doses until the desired response is obtained (usual maximum dose, 1 g). The usual daily maintenance dose is 400 to 800 mg (15 to 30 mg/kg); the frequency of administration must be individualized. For children 4 to 6 years, 10 to 20 mg/kg in two or three divided doses is warranted, increased by up to 100 mg daily at weekly intervals, as needed and tolerated. The usual maintenance dose is 250 to 350 mg a day (usual maximum dose, 400 mg). For children under 4 years, an initial dose of 20 to 60 mg is recommended.[7]

For adults and adolescents, initially 400 mg should be divided into two doses on the first day, increased by 200 mg daily at appropriate intervals (usually 1 to 2 weeks) and administered in three or four divided doses. The usual daily maintenance dose is 600 mg to 1.2 g in monotherapy, but may be as high as 2.0 g in combination therapy.

Although extensive studies are not available, it appears that elderly patients metabolize carbamazepine more slowly and therefore will need lower doses.

Generic: tablets 200 mg; chewable tablets 100 mg.

Tegretol (Basel): tablets 200 mg; chewable tablets 100 mg; suspension 100 mg/5 mL.

Adverse Reactions and Precautions

Baseline blood and platelet counts, urinalysis, and hepatic and renal function studies should be performed before initiating treatment with carbamazepine. But excessively frequent and specialized monitoring is unwarranted and costly. Careful attention to new symptoms is probably equally effective in preventing serious complications.[8] Blood counts should be performed once or twice during the first few months of therapy as part of the routine monitoring of plasma drug concentrations, and then only periodically thereafter if no abnormalities appear. Dermatologic reactions such as pruritic and erythematous rashes and urticaria have been reported in 2% to 4% of patients. Less common but more serious are Stevens-Johnson syndrome, photosensitivity, exfoliative dermatitis, erythema multiforme, erythema nodosum, and aggravation of systemic lupus erythematosus. Petechiae, pallor, weakness, fever, or infection may be symptoms of a potentially fatal reaction and patients should be instructed to contact their physician immediately.

Less serious side effects that occur during early treatment with carbamazepine are drowsiness, dizziness, lightheadedness, diplopia, ataxia, nausea, and vomiting. These usually subside spontaneously within a week or after a reduction in dose. Less common neurologic reactions include confusion, headache, fatigue, blurred vision, oculomotor disturbances, dysphasia, abnormal involuntary movements, peripheral neuritis and paresthesias, depression with agitation, talkativeness, nystagmus, and tinnitus.

Gastrointestinal reactions include gastric distress and abdominal pain, diarrhea, constipation, and anorexia. Dryness of the mouth, glossitis, and stomatitis also occur.

Transient leukopenia occurs in approximately 10% of patients treated with carbamazepine, but discontinuance of the drug usually is not required. Other hematopoietic reactions (eosinophilia, leukocytosis, purpura, and thrombocytopenia) are rare. Although very uncommon, these reactions may be fatal. Because their onset is gradual and reversible when the drug is discontinued, patients should be advised to notify their physician if fever, sore throat, aphthous stomatitis, easy bruising, petechial or purpuric hemorrhage, or other signs of hematologic toxicity appear.

Carbamazepine has an antidiuretic hormonelike effect that may be troublesome, particularly in cardiac or elderly patients. Mild, asymptomatic hyponatremia is a common laboratory finding.[9] Serious water intoxication with sodium concentrations below 120 mEq/L—and characterized by confusion, lethargy, neurologic dysfunction, and seizures—is uncommon. The risk increases with age (all cases have been reported in adults or elderly) and with elevated carbamazepine plasma concentrations. Other drugs predisposing to water intoxication should be avoided when carbamazepine is used.

Cardiovascular, genitourinary, metabolic, hepatic, and other reactions have been reported rarely. These include aggravation of hypertension or ischemic heart disease, arrhythmias, hypotension, syncope, edema, congestive heart failure, recurrence of thrombophlebitis, urinary frequency, acute urinary retention, albuminuria, glycosuria, elevated blood urea nitrogen levels, microscopic deposits in the urine, impotence, cholestatic and hepatocellular jaundice, fever and chills, myalgia and arthralgia, leg cramps, and conjunctivitis.

Drug Interactions

Approximately 75% of carbamazepine is bound to plasma albumin, but it is not significantly displaced by other drugs. As a result of enzyme induction, carbamazepine increases the hepatic metabolism of clonazepam, diazepam, ethosuximide, and valproate. In patients treated with phenobarbital, phenytoin, or primidone concomitantly, a small increase or, more commonly, a decrease in the plasma concentration of one or both agents may occur. Likewise, valproate has a variable effect on carbamazepine steady-state concentrations and decreases carbamazepine epoxide metabolism, which may have therapeutic or toxic significance.[6]

Carbamazepine concentrations are markedly increased by erythromycin and propoxyphene hydrochloride. Cimetidine, danazol, diltiazem, isoniazid, propoxyphene, troleandomycin, and verapamil also increase the plasma concentration of carbamazepine, but to a lesser degree. The effect of cimetidine is transient. In pediatric patients, large doses of nicotinamide may increase carbamazepine plasma concentrations. Carbamazepine increases the hepatic clearance and may decrease the effectiveness of oral anticoagulants, certain anti-infectives (doxycycline, mebendazole) haloperidol, and theophylline. Carbamazepine also may reduce the plasma concentration and therapeutic response to corticosteroids or thyroid hormones. Other drug interactions (eg, with quinidine, oral contraceptives) related to hepatic enzyme induction that have been reported for other antiepileptic drugs conceivably could occur with carbamazepine but are not well documented. The combination of carbamazepine and lithium may increase the risk of neurotoxicity.

Phenytoin: Actions and Uses

Phenytoin (Dilantin®) is useful in generalized tonic-clonic, complex partial, and simple partial seizures. Comparative data from clinical trials indicate that phenytoin is better tolerated than phenobarbital and primidone.[5] It is ineffective in absence, myoclonic, and atonic seizures and is not recommended for the treatment of epileptic syndromes in which absence seizures or myoclonus are present. Intravenous phenytoin sodium is an effective treatment for status epilepticus and can be used as the initial drug to manage recurrent seizures.

Pharmacokinetics

Bioavailability of phenytoin averages 85% to 90% with most preparations. Time to peak plasma concentration is variable and increases with the dose, but normally occurs within 4 to 8 hours for prompt-release capsules, and somewhat later for the extended-release preparations. Plasma protein binding is 90%. Phenytoin is eliminated almost entirely by hepatic metabolism. Oxidative metabolism proceeds via an epoxide intermediate, which probably represents the rate-limiting step.

Plasma concentrations are not related linearly to the daily dose because of saturable nonlinear metabolism, and small increases in dose may greatly increase the plasma concentration. Plasma concentrations of

10 to 20 mg/L are usually effective. However, higher or lower concentrations may sometimes be therapeutic and clinical outcome should determine the appropriate level for each patient.

Since phenytoin demonstrates nonlinear elimination kinetics, clearance and apparent half-life are dose-dependent. However, there is significant intersubject variability in phenytoin metabolism. Methods used to guide phenytoin dose adjustments include: graphic, which employs a linear transformation of the Michaelis-Menten equation; nomograms; estimates using population clearance values; and bayesian procedures. A simple method using a semilogarithmic plot of steady-state drug concentrations versus corresponding maintenance doses also has been described.[10]

Phenytoin's nonlinear kinetics accentuate the variations in blood levels caused by alterations in the rates of dissolution and absorption among the various dosage forms and products. Thus, phenytoin plasma concentrations may differ significantly from one product to another.[11]

The plasma concentration of free phenytoin can be increased by hyperbilirubinemia (eg, in neonates, in those with liver disease), hypoalbuminemia (eg, in the elderly, in those with liver disease), and uremia. Febrile illnesses may markedly increase the clearance of phenytoin, leading to lowered plasma concentrations.[12] Phenytoin plasma concentrations also may be reduced by concurrent enteral feeding.[13]

Dosage and Preparations

Oral: The dosage must be individualized according to the patient's response and to the drug concentrations. Phenytoin may be administerd in divided doses (but does not need to be dosed more than twice daily). In adults, once-daily administration is usually sufficient to maintain plasma concentrations in the therapeutic range once steady state has been achieved. It also improves compliance. However, once-daily dosage may not be practical in patients who tend to miss doses.

For adults, initially 300 mg daily is recommended in two divided doses; the maintenance dose is usually 300 to 400 mg or 4 to 6 mg/kg/day. Incremental increases can be made using 30-mg capsules; 50-mg chewable tablets are also available. Formulation differences between tablet and capsules may cause problems in precise dose titration. The tablets (free acid phenytoin) contain 8% more phenytoin than the phenytoin sodium capsules.

Dosing regimens for the elderly have not been well established but are usually 3 to 4 mg/kg/day lower than those in adults.

For children, initially 5 mg/kg/day is recommended in two divided doses, with the maintenance dose individualized. Maintenance doses may need to be higher, 7 mg/kg/day or more.

Intravenous: Phenytoin is very water insoluble. The present preparation is 40% propylene glycol, 10% alcohol, and adjusted to a pH of 12. It must be administered slowly to avoid hypotension or cardiac arrhythmias. Also, it is very sclerosing, and must be given through an intracatheter into a large vein. If given into a small hand or forearm vein, it will be quite painful and cause venous sclerosis, "the purple hand." Leakage from the injection site into the subcutaneous tissue can cause necrosis. To circumvent these problems, a prodrug has been developed, fosphenytoin. It consists of a phosphate group that is joined to the phenytoin molecule by an ester bond (Figure 2). This molecule is rapidly and completely converted in vivo to phenytoin with a half-life of 8 to 12 minutes. Thus, within 20 to 30 minutes, almost all of the fosphenytoin has been converted to phenytoin in the body. The advantages of this preparation are that it is formulated in aqueous solution near normal pH and without propylene glycol or alcohol. It is well tolerated and does not cause venous sclerosis. Also, it can be administered without the complications associated with the present preparation.[14] When fosphenytoin is available in 1996, it should completely replace the present formulation, primarily because of safety considerations.

Intramuscular: The phenytoin preparation now in use should not be given intramuscularly because it precipitates, forming painful and insoluble crystals. The absorption rate is erratic. The new preparation, fosphenytoin, is readily absorbed after IM injection. It causes little discomfort.[14] The availability of this IM preparation will make it possible to replace oral phenytoin in situations where a patient is NPO without resorting to IV administration. Also, this preparation may be used when a patient has had some seizures and has a low phenytoin level. The situation may not be urgent enough to require IV loading, but the oral preparation does not reach peak absorption for 8 to 12 hours. The use of fosphenytoin IM would be useful in this situation.

Phenytoin (free acid):

Generic: Suspension 125 mg/

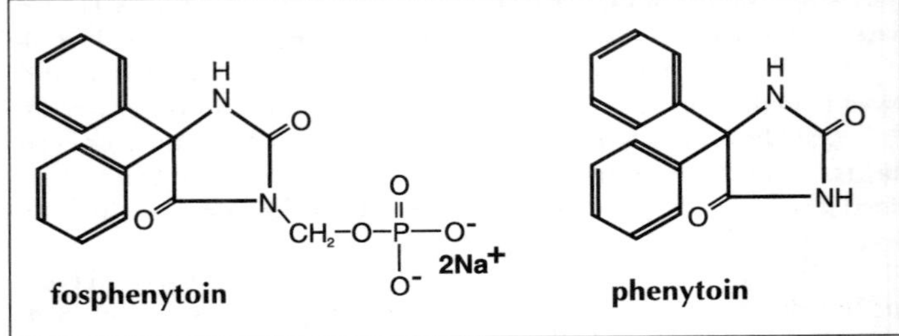

Figure 2*—Chemical formulae for fosphenytoin and for phenytoin.*

5 mL (alcohol < 0.6%).

Dilantin (Parke-Davis): Suspension 125 mg/5 mL (alcohol < 0.6%); tablets (chewable) 50 mg.

Phenytoin sodium:

Generic: Capsules (prompt) 100 mg.

Dilantin (Parke-Davis). Capsules (extended) 30 mg and 100 mg.

Phenytoin solution:

Generic: Solution 50 mg/mL in propylene glycol 40%, alcohol 10%, pH adjusted to 11-12.

Dilantin (Parke-Davis). This preparation will be discontinued in 1996 and replaced by Cerebyx®.

Fosphenytoin solution:

Cerebyx 75 mg/mL (equivalent to 50 mg/mL of phenytoin) in 2-mL and 5-mL vials.

Adverse Reactions and Precautions

Phenytoin produces little or no sedation at concentrations below 20 mg/L. Plasma concentrations above 20 mg/L may be associated with concentration-dependent symptoms of toxicity: nystagmus, ataxia, and lethargy. However, in the absence of symptoms, doses should not be decreased if needed for control of seizures.

Skin eruptions occur in approximately 8% of patients but are rarely serious and are unrelated to the initial dosage or to the plasma concentration.[15] Peripheral neuropathy may develop after years of use. Mild gingival hyperplasia may be seen on careful oral examinations in 20% to 50% of patients. Scrupulous oral hygiene prevents secondary inflammation and severe hyperplasia is uncommon. Hypertrichosis and hirsutism are less common.

Rare but serious idiosyncratic reactions include hepatitis, bone-marrow depression, systemic lupus erythematosus, Stevens-Johnson syndrome, and lymphadenopathy. These often disappear after therapy is discontinued. A few cases of lymphoma and Hodgkin's disease have been reported.

Drug Interactions

Phenytoin may reduce the plasma concentration of carbamazepine, valproate, ethosuximide, and primidone by enzyme induction. Phenytoin and phenobarbital exert variable, reciprocal effects. Valproate displaces phenytoin from protein-binding sites but inhibits metabolism. Total plasma concentrations may be decreased, but the unbound (free) may change little or may increase.

Other drugs that may displace phenytoin include phenylbutazone, salicylates, and tolbutamide. The total plasma concentration of phenytoin may decrease, but the actual free concentration may be relatively unchanged because of the increase in the free fraction. Drugs that significantly increase the plasma concentration of phenytoin include chloramphenicol, cimetidine, dicumarol, disulfiram, isoniazid, sulfonamides, and trimethoprim. Amiodarone, allopurinol, chlorpheniramine, and trazodone may possibly increase the plasma phenytoin concentration. Folic acid, prolonged ingestion of alcohol, and rifampin may decrease the phenytoin plasma concentration. In patients with tuberculosis, the effects of rifampin and isoniazid may cancel each other when these drugs are used with phenytoin. Certain antineoplastic agents (bleomycin, cisplatin, vinblastine) may also reduce plasma concentrations of phenytoin.

Phenytoin is a relatively potent enzyme inducer and may decrease the effectiveness of oral anticoagulants, certain antibiotics (doxycycline, rifampin, and chloramphenicol), oral contraceptives, antiarrhythmic agents (disopyramide, mexiletine, quinidine) digitoxin, analgesics (meperidine, methadone), cyclosporine, corticosteroids, and theophylline. Pharmacologically, phenytoin has been reported to impair blood pressure control by dopamine and to decrease the response to nondepolarizing skeletal muscle relaxants.

Valproate: Actions and Uses

Valproate (valproic acid [Depakene®] and divalproex sodium [Depakote®]) control absence, myoclonic, and tonic seizures in generalized, idiopathic epilepsy. It is most useful in typical absence seizures. Valproate is as effective as ethosuximide in patients with absence seizures alone and is variably effective in atypical absence seizures. Valproate is the drug of choice for patients with both absence and generalized tonic-clonic seizures.

The precise role of valproate in the treatment of partial seizures remains to be established. Retrospective comparisons of valproate with carbamazepine or phenytoin in the treatment of partial and secondarily generalized seizures indicate that valproate is equally effective. But a prospective, controlled multicenter trial of carbamazepine and valproate in partial seizures indicated carbamazepine to be slightly more effective.[16]

Valproate is the drug of choice in myoclonic epilepsy, with or without generalized tonic-clonic seizures that begin in adolescence or early adulthood. Valproate usually controls photosensitive myoclonus and is also effective in the treatment of benign myoclonic epilepsy, postanoxic myoclonus, and, with clonazepam, in severe progressive myoclonic epilepsy that is characterized by tonic-clonic seizures. It also may be preferred in certain stimulus-sensitive (reflex, startle) epilepsies.

Although valproate may be effective for infantile spasms, it is relatively contraindicated in children whose spasms are caused by hyperglycinemia or other underlying metabolic (mitochondrial) abnormalities.

In general, atonic and akinetic seizures in patients with Lennox-Gastaut syndrome are difficult to control, but valproate is an effective drug of choice for treatment of these mixed seizure types.

Because valproate has been useful in many patients who are refractory to other antiepileptic drugs, it may warrant a trial in nonresponsive patients regardless of seizure type.

Pharmacokinetics

Valproic acid (Depakene) is absorbed rapidly and completely in the stomach after oral administration; peak plasma concentrations usually occur within 0.5 to 2 hours. The delayed-release tablet preparation, divalproex sodium (Depakote), reaches peak plasma concentrations 3 to 6 hours after ingestion. Although absorption is delayed, its total availability is unaffected by food.

The plasma protein binding of valproate is saturable within the usual therapeutic range (approximately 90% at 75 mg/L). Usual effective plasma concentrations range from 50 to 100 mg/L, but higher concentrations exceeding 150 mg/L may be required and tolerated in some patients. With a daily dose of more than 50 mg/kg, plasma concentrations may not increase proportionately because both clearance and free fraction increase. Daily fluctuations in free fraction and clearance also occur as a result of displacement by free fatty acids or circadian influences. Thus, when plasma concentrations are being monitored, samples should be taken at a uniform time.

Valproate is eliminated almost exclusively by hepatic metabolism. Its metabolic fate is complex. A variety of conjugation and oxidative processes are involved, including pathways (eg, beta oxidation) normally reserved for endogenous fatty acids. As the dose is increased, mitochondrial beta oxidation occurs. In mitochondrial pathways, sequential use of acetyl-CoA and carnitine may interfere with intermediary metabolism. Rarely, valproate may induce secondary carnitine deficiency.

Metabolites may contribute to both antiepileptic and hepatotoxic effects. The antiepileptic activity of valproate (including the time course) is poorly correlated with steady-state valproate plasma concentrations. This may be due to the fact that one metabolite, the 2-ene-VPA, has antiepileptic properties. Another metabolite, 2-n-propyl-4-pentenoic acid (4-ene-VPA), has been proposed as a key hepatotoxic metabolite.

The half-life of valproate in adults is 12 to 16 hours. In epileptic patients receiving polytherapy, the half-life is shorter, approximately 9 hours or less in school-age children and young adolescents. Elimination half-lives of valproate are longer in neonates and generally shorter during middle and late infancy. Because hepatic clearance is reduced, the drug's half-life in geriatric patients is approximately 15 hours. Also, because of lower albumin concentrations, the free fraction may be higher in this group.

Dosage and Preparations

Oral: Adults, initially 5 to 15 mg/kg/day; usual maintenance dose, 15 to 25 mg/kg/day.

When used with other antiepileptic drugs, the initial dose is 10 to 30 mg/kg/day, and the usual maintenance dose is 30 to 60 mg/kg/day.

Children 1 to 12 years, initially, 10 to 30 mg/kg/day; maintenance dose 20 to 30 mg/kg/day. When used with other antiepileptic drugs that induce hepatic metabolism, the initial dose is 15 to 45 mg/kg/day and the usual maintenance dose is 30 to 100 mg/kg/day. With polytherapy, some pediatric patients may require more than 100 mg/kg/day to establish therapeutic plasma concentrations. Depakote Sprinkle may be preferable for use in children and elderly patients because it is more palatable than the syrup, can be sprinkled over food, and is slowly absorbed, which may reduce fluctuations in concentrations.

Dosing regimens for the elderly have not been well established, but lower doses may be needed because of slower hepatic metabolism.

Valproic Acid:

Generic: capsules 250 mg

Depakene (Abbott), capsules 250 mg; syrup 250 mg/5 mL

Divalproex Sodium:

Depakote (Abbott), tablets (delayed-release) 125, 250, and 500 mg.

Depakote Sprinkle (Abbott), capsules 125 mg.

Adverse Reactions and Precautions

Adverse reactions generally appear early in the course of therapy and are mild and transient.

The incidence of gastrointestinal disturbances (nausea, vomiting, anorexia, heartburn) ranges from 6% to 45%. Symptoms are transient and rarely require drug withdrawal. Gastrointenstinal discomfort may be diminished by administering the delayed-release preparation (Depakote or Depakote Sprinkle). Diarrhea, abdominal cramps, and constipation are reported occasionally. Increased appetite with weight gain is common and may be controlled by diet, but in some cases, excessive weight gain may require withdrawal of valproate.

Hand tremor, similar to benign essential tremor, is the most common neurologic side effect and occasionally is severe enough to interfere with writing. Tremor occurs more frequently with high doses and may improve with a reduction in dosage.

Sedation and drowsiness develop infrequently in patients receiving valproate alone. Conversely, central nervous system stimulation and excitement have been observed, and aggressiveness and hyperactivity are sometimes noted in children. Ataxia, headache, and stupor have been reported rarely.

Alopecia, thinning, or changes in hair texture occur in some patients, but these effects usually are temporary and do not require the withdrawal of the drug. Rash occurs rarely.

Valproate inhibits the secondary phase of platelet aggregation, but this is usually not clinically significant. But patients should not receive other drugs that affect coagulation. Thrombocytopenia has been observed, but its incidence is not known. Rarely, hematomas, epistaxis, and increased bleeding after surgery have been reported and platelet function should be monitored before surgery.

A few cases of severe or fatal pancreatitis have been reported. This complication is accompanied by severe abdominal pain, vomiting, and elevated amylase.

Transient elevations of liver transaminases (eg, aspartate aminotransferase [AST]) are common. The elevations usually are not related to serious liver dysfunction, and levels often return to normal with or without dosage adjustment. However, fatal hepatotoxicity has occurred during valproate therapy. Prodromal illness characterized by muscle weakness, lethargy, anorexia, and vomiting is often present. Hepatotoxicity usually develops after an average of 2 months (range, 3 days to 6 months) of therapy.

In the United States, 37 fatalities associated with valproate were reported between 1978 and 1984. Most occurred in children receiving polytherapy and in patients with mental retardation, congenital abnormalities, or other neurologic diseases. Based on retrospective analyses, the following risks for fatal hepatotoxicity from valproate were identified: overall, 1:10,000; polytherapy: children <2 years, 1:500; >2 years, 1:12,000; monotherapy: overall, 1:37,000; children <2 years, 1:7,000; >2 years, 1:45,000.[17]

Since 1984, hepatic fatalities associated with the use of valproate have decreased. During 1985 and 1986, five fatalities (none in individuals over 10 years of age) among 198,000 patients were reported (incidence, 1:49,000). This can be attributed to a change in the prescribing patterns for valproate, including increased use of monotherapy and decreased use in high-risk patients.[17]

Guidelines for valproate recommended by the American Academy of Pediatrics and others include:

(1) Avoid administering valproate as polytherapy in children under 3 years of age unless monotherapy has failed to control seizures.

(2) Use other effective therapy initially when possible (eg, in absence and febrile seizures), although valproate is effective in many of these and other types of seizures.

(3) Avoid administering valproate to patients with preexisting hepatic disease or with family history of childhood hepatic disease or to critically ill children and children receiving other medication that affects coagulation.

(4) Assess liver function before therapy, 3 to 5 weeks after initiation of treatment, approxi-

mately monthly during the first 6 months of use, and periodically thereafter.

(5) Instruct patients and their parents to report symptoms, such as loss of appetite, lethargy, nausea, vomiting, abdominal pain, jaundice, edema, easy bruising, and loss of seizure control, because laboratory monitoring alone may be inadequate to diagnose valproate-induced hepatotoxicity. However, if laboratory tests indicate clinically important hepatic dysfunction, discontinuation of the drug should be considered.

(6) Maintain dosage at the lowest amount that produces optimal seizure control. Routine monitoring of liver function does not always detect hepatotoxicity of rapid onset, since it may not be preceded by elevation of AST.

Valproate therapy commonly produces reversible hyperammonemia, but there does not appear to be any clinical significance to this reaction in the absence of liver dysfunction.

Drug Reactions

Valproate inhibits phenobarbital metabolism and the plasma phenobarbital concentration may increase by 25% to 68% when valproate is added.[18] This can cause marked sedation or intoxication attributable to phenobarbital. Therefore, a 30% to 75% reduction in phenobarbital dosage is required when valproate is added to the regimen, and 2 to 3 weeks must elapse before a new steady-state level is achieved.

The interaction between valproate and phenytoin is complex. Valproate displaces phenytoin from plasma albumin, which temporarily increases the ratio of free/bound drug; toxicity may result if phenytoin concentrations were high before administration of valproate. The total phenytoin plasma concentration may decrease by about 30% during the first several weeks of therapy, but usually does not result in recurrence of seizures because the free phenytoin concentration does not change. However, valproate also may inhibit the biotransformation of phenytoin, which, over the next 4 to 16 weeks, produces a gradual return of total phenytoin plasma concentrations to previous values. Measurement of unbound phenytoin concentration may be useful as a means of explaining the onset of central nervous system toxicity when the total plasma phenytoin concentration is within the therapeutic range.

Valproate displaces diazepam from protein-binding sites and may augment its sedative action.

Other interactions between valproate and phenobarbital,

primidone, phenytoin, and carbamazepine result from the enzyme-inducing effects of the latter drugs, which reduce the half-life of valproate. The half-life of valproate is not consistently affected by ethosuximide or the benzodiazepines. Valproate does not induce liver enzymes. It increases the concentration of carbamazepine epoxide by blocking epoxide hydrolase. In some patients, aspirin or other salicylates may displace valproate from protein-binding sites and cause a sufficient increase in unbound valproate concentrations to result in toxicity.

Clonazepam: Actions and Uses

Clonazepam (Klonopin®) may be useful alone or in combination with other drugs to control myoclonic or atonic seizures and photosensitive epilepsy. In patients with juvenile myoclonic epilepsy, clonazepam may help control myoclonic jerks but it has not been shown to be useful for the treatment of generalized tonic-clonic seizures.[19]

Pharmacokinetics

Clonazepam is well absorbed; peak plasma concentrations occur 1 to 4 hours after oral administration. It is almost completely biotransformed to inactive metabolites. The reported half-life ranges are similar for adults (19 to 50 hours) and children (22 to 33 hours).

Dosage and Preparations

Oral: Adults, initially 1.5 mg daily in three divided doses, increased by 0.5 to 1 mg every third day until seizures are adequately controlled or until adverse effects occur.

Children, doses of 0.5 mg should be used initially.

Doses for the elderly have not been well established.

Klonopin (Roche), tablets 0.5, 1, and 2 mg.

Adverse Reactions and Precautions

The most common adverse effects of clonazepam involve the central nervous system. Approximately one half of patients experience drowsiness, about one third ataxia, and up to one quarter personality changes. The sedation may be minimized by initiating therapy with a small dose and increasing the amount gradually.

Drug Interactions

Interactions between clonazepam and other antiepileptic drugs usually are not significant.

Diazepam: Actions and Uses

Intravenous diazepam (Valium®) is effective in continuous tonic-clonic status epilepticus. Its duration of action is short because of its rapid redistribution from the brain. A loading dose of intravenous phenytoin sodium should be given concomitantly or immediately after control of seizures is achieved with diazepam to maintain antiepileptic activity. Maintenance therapy with oral diazepam is usually not useful in treating epilepsy.

Rectal administration of the parenteral solution of diazepam is effective for the short-term prophylaxis of febrile seizures.[20]

Pharmacokinetics

Diazepam's onset of action is almost immediate after intravenous administration. The volume of distribution is reported to be 0.95 to 2 L/kg. The half-lives of diazepam and its active derivative, desmethyldiazepam, are 27 to 37, and 50 to 100 hours, respectively; however, rapid redistribution from the brain occurs within 30 minutes after injection.

Dosage and Preparations

Intravenous: Adults, 5 to 10 mg initially; then as needed to control seizures.

Intravenous: Children, 0.5 mg, followed by 0.25 mg/kg as needed.

Intravenous: Elderly, 5 mg cautiously, with subsequent doses based on the patient's response.

Rectally: Children, 0.5 to 0.8 mg for children under 3 years of age; 0.6 to 0.9 mg for children over 3 years of age.

Generic: solution 5 mg/mL in 1-mL, 2-mL, and 10-mL containers.

Valium (Roche), solution 5 mg/mL in 2-mL and 10-mL containers.

Adverse Reactions and Precautions

When diazepam is administered parenterally for the treatment of status epilepticus, the patient must be observed for signs of respiratory and central nervous system depression and hypotension. This is especially true when diazepam is administered with other antiepileptic agents.

Ethosuximide: Actions and Uses

Ethosuximide (Zarontin®) is the drug of choice for absence seizures unaccompanied by other types of seizures. Ethosuximide is preferred to other succinimides because it is more effective and less likely to produce drowsiness and gastrointestinal upset than its chemical relatives.

Ethosuximide also may be effective in myoclonic seizures and akinetic epilepsy, but it is generally ineffective in complex partial or generalized tonic-clonic seizures.

Pharmacokinetics

Ethosuximide is well absorbed orally, and the peak plasma concentration occurs in 1 to 4 hours. It is minimally bound to plasma protein and eliminated primarily via hepatic metabolism, with 10% to 20% of the administered dose excreted unchanged in the urine. The half-life is variable but averages 52 to 56 hours in adults and 32 to 41 hours in children. Control of absence seizures usually is achieved with plasma concentrations of 40 to 100 mg/L, but higher concentrations may be required and tolerated.

Dosage and Preparations

Oral: Adults and children over 6 years of age, initially 500 mg daily, increased if necessary by 250 mg every 4 to 7 days until seizures are controlled or until untoward effects develop. The daily maintenance dose is usually 15 to 40 mg/kg.

Children 3 to 6 years of age, initially 250 mg daily with incremental increases in dosage, as for older patients. The daily maintenance dose is usually 15 to 40 mg/kg.

Zarontin (Parke-Davis), capsules 250 mg; syrup 250 mg/5 mL.

Adverse Reactions and Precautions

The most common adverse reactions to ethosuximide are gastrointestinal disturbances (eg, nausea, vomiting).

Drug Interactions

Ethosuximide does not consistently alter the plasma concentration of other antiepileptic drugs.

Phenobarbital: Actions and Uses

Phenobarbital (phenobarbital sodium), a long-acting barbiturate, is effective in generalized tonic-clonic and simple partial seizures. Phenobarbital frequently is used to treat neonatal seizures and may be the initial drug employed in young children. However, because of increasing concern about adverse neuropsychologic reactions to sedative/hypnotic antiepileptic drugs, many clinicians prefer less sedating drugs.

Pharmacokinetics

Phenobarbital is almost completely absorbed orally, but 1 to 6 hours may be necessary to achieve peak plasma concentrations. The drug also is well absorbed after intramuscular injection. Protein binding is about 45% in adults. The average plasma half-life is 3 days in children and 4 days in adults; consequently, 3 or more weeks may be required to attain steady-state plasma concentrations.

Plasma concentrations of 15 to 40 mg/L are usually optimal

for the control of epilepsy.

Phenobarbital: Dosage and Preparations

Oral: Adults, 120 to 250 mg; alternatively, 2 to 3 mg/kg/day. The elderly may need lower doses. Children, 30 to 100 mg daily; these amounts are taken at bedtime. Administration more than once a day is unnecessary.

Generic: elixir 15 and 20 mg/mL; tablets 8, 15, 30, 60, and 100 mg.

Adverse Reactions and Precautions

Although phenobarbital is associated with significant behavioral and subtle cognitive effects, it may cause less toxicity (hematopoietic, hepatic) than the other drugs. Drowsiness is the most common adverse reaction, although tolerance usually develops and a significant percentage of patients continue to experience sedation. Furthermore, phenobarbital may affect memory, perceptual motor performance, and tasks requiring sustained performance. Phenobarbital markedly influences behavior; it can provoke irritability and exacerbate existing behavioral problems, particularly hyperkinesia.

A substantial number of adults who take phenobarbital develop depression. An occasional patient may become excitable; children and the elderly are most susceptible. Phenobarbital must be used cautiously in the elderly because of its propensity to cause sedation, depression, and mental slowing. These side effects may either exacerbate existing symptoms of declining brain function or may be confused for the onset of dementia. Abrupt termination of therapy may exacerbate seizures, but drug dependence is unlikely with usual antiepileptic doses. Skin eruptions are uncommon.

Drug Interactions

Phenobarbital both induces hepatic enzymes and competitively inhibits drug biotransformation. Thus, mutual enzyme induction or inhibition in patients treated with phenobarbital and phenytoin may result in an increase, decrease, or no change in the plasma concentration of one or both of the drugs.

Because it induces hepatic enzymes, phenobarbital may enhance the hepatic clearance and decrease the clinical effectiveness of oral anticoagulants, oral contraceptives, anti-infectives (chloramphenicol, doxycycline, griseofulvin), lipophilic betablockers (eg, propranolol, metoprolol), corticosteroids, cyclosporine, tricyclic antidepressants (eg, desipramine, nortriptyline), haloperidol, phenothiazines, quinidine, theophylline, digitoxin, doxorubicin, and verapamil.

Primidone: Actions and Uses

Primidone is a deoxybarbiturate (Mysoline®) closely related chemically to the barbiturates. It is converted to two active metabolites, phenobarbital and phenylethylmalonamide (PEMA). Primidone is used principally in generalized tonic-clonic and complex and simple partial seizures. It is as effective as carbamazepine or phenytoin in controlling partial or generalized tonic-clonic seizures, although its greater incidence of adverse reactions limits patient acceptance.[5]

Pharmacokinetics

Primidone is rapidly and completely absorbed after oral administration; peak plasma concentrations are attained in an average of 4 hours, but there is wide interpatient variation. Primidone is metabolized to phenobarbital and PEMA, but a considerable percentage of the administered dose is excreted unchanged. Because the half-life of primidone (9 to 22 hours) is considerably shorter than that of phenobarbital, plasma concentrations of phenobarbital are generally higher than that of primidone. Phenobarbital concentrations should be measured when monitoring primidone therapy.

Dosage and Preparations

Oral: Adults and older children, initially 125 mg at bedtime for 3 days, with the dose increased by 125 mg every 3 days until a maintenance dose of 250 mg 3 times a day is established on the 10th day. The amount may be adjusted to a maximum of 2 g/day administered in three or four divided doses. The elderly may need lower doses.

Children under 8 years of age, initially one half of the adult dosage. For maintenance, 125 mg to 250 mg is given 3 times a day.

Generic: tablets 250 mg

Mysoline (Wyeth-Ayerst), suspension 250 mg/5 mL; tablets 50 and 250 mg.

Adverse Reactions and Precautions

Sedation is common but often diminishes with continued administration.

Infrequently Used AEDs

Acetazolamide (Ak-Zol®, Diamox®), a carbonic anhydrase inhibitor, has been used in absence, generalized tonic-clonic, and partial seizures. It is most often administered as an adjunct to other drugs, but its usefulness is limited by the rapid development of tolerance in some patients. Acetazolamide is most widely used intermittently in women whose seizure frequency increases with menstruation.

Dosage and Preparations

Oral: Adults and children, 8 to 30 mg/kg daily in divided doses (range, 250 mg to 1 g daily).

Generic: tablets 250 mg

Ak-Zol (Akorn), tablets 250 mg.

References

1. Federal Food, Drug, and Cosmetic Act of 1938, Public Law 717, 75th Congress.

2. Merritt HH, Putnam TJ: Sodium diphenylhydantoinate in the treatment of convulsive disorders. *JAMA* 1938;111: 1068-1073.

3. Leppik IE: Compliance during the treatment of epilepsy. *Epilepsia* 1988;29(suppl 2):S79-S84.

4. Snead OC III, Hosey LC: Exacerbation of seizures in children by carbamazepine. *N Engl J Med* 1985;313:916-921.

5. Mattson RH, et al: Comparison of carbamazepine, phenobarbital, phenytoin, and primidone in partial and secondarily generalized tonic-clonic seizures. *N Engl J Med* 1985;313:145-151.

6. Bourgeois BFD, Wad NL: Individualized and combined antiepileptic and neurotoxic activity of carbamazepine and carbamazepine-10,11-epoxide in mice. *J Pharmacol Exp Ther* 1984;231:411-415.

7. Porter RJ: How to initiate and maintain carbamazepine therapy in children and adults. *Epilepsia* 1987;28(suppl 3):S59-S63.

8. Pellock JM: Carbamazepine side effects in children and adults. *Epilepsia* 1987; 28(suppl 3):S64-S70.

9. Lahr MB: Hyponatremia during carbamazepine therapy. *Clin Pharmacol Ther* 1985; 37:693-696.

10. Wagner JG: New and simple method to predict dosage of drugs obeying simple Michaelis-Menten elimination kinetics and to distinguish such kinetics from simple first order and from parallel Michaelis-Menten and first order kinetics. *Ther Drug Monit* 1985;7:377-386.

11. Nuwer MR, Browne TR, Dodson WE, et al: Generic substitutions for antiepileptic drugs. *Neurology* 1990;40:1647-1651.

12. Leppik IE, Fisher J, Kriel R, et al: Altered phenytoin clearance during febrile illness. *Neurology* 1986;36:1367-1370.

13. Haley CJ, Nelson J: Phenytoin-enteral feeding interaction. *Ann Pharmacother* 1989; 23:796-798.

14. Leppik IE, Boucher BA, Wilder BJ, et al: Pharmacokinetics and safety of a phenytoin prodrug given IV or IM in patients. *Neurology* 1990;40: 456-460.

15. Leppik IE, Lapora J, Lowenson R, et al: Seasonal in-

cidence of phenytoin allergy unrelated to plasma levels. *Arch Neurol* 1985;42:120-122.

16. Mattson RH, Cramer JA, Collins JF, et al: Valproate vs carbamazepine for seizures, a comparison of valproate with carbamazepine for the treatment of complex partial seizures and secondarily generalized tonic-clonic seizures in adults. *N Engl J Med* 1992; 327(11):765.

17. Dreifuss FE, Santilli N, Langer DH, et al: Valproic acid hepatic fatalities: a retrospective review. *Neurology* 1987; 37:379-385.

18. Richens A, Ahmad S: Controlled trial of sodium valproate in severe epilepsy. *Br Med J* 1975;4:255-256.

19. Obeid T, Panayiotopoulos CP: Clonazepam in juvenile myoclonic epilepsy. *Epilepsia* 1989;30:603-606.

20. Knudsen FU: Effective short-term diazepam prophylaxis in febrile convulsions. *J Pediatr* 1985;106:487-490.

Chapter 8

Newly Approved Antiepileptic Drugs

Before 1993, the last major drug that the FDA approved for epilepsy was valproate, in 1978. During the 1970s, the Epilepsy Branch of the National Institutes of Health (NIH) recognized the need for new antiepileptic drugs and implemented a comprehensive system for screening promising compounds in animal models of epilepsy. Since then, more than 17,000 compounds have been evaluated.

Those meeting strict standards of effectiveness and safety have been entered into clinical trials. They have been tested principally for activity against complex partial seizures with or without secondary generalization in adults. Felbamate has been studied in the Lennox-Gastaut syndrome in children. Some persons under age 18 have been included in these studies.

Now the efforts of more

Table 1
New Antiepileptic Drugs Available in 1996

Name	Approved Daily Dose	Half-Life	Significant Drug Interactions
Gabapentin (Neurontin®)	900-1800 mg* in adults	4-6 hr	None
Lamotrigine (Lamictal®)	150-600 mg in adults	15-24 hr	Valproate increases lamotrigine levels
Felbamate (Felbatol®)	1800-3600 mg+ in adults; 15-45 mg/kg in children	15-24 hr	Felbamate increases phenytoin and valproate levels

* Doses as high as 4800 mg/d have been used and 2400 to 3600 mg/d are well tolerated.

\+ Doses up to 5200 mg/d have been used.

than a decade of preclinical and clinical testing are bearing fruit. The FDA approved felbamate and gabapentin in 1993 and lamotrigine in 1994 (Table 1). All three new drugs are now available by prescription.

Because of reports of aplastic anemia associated with the use of felbamate, the FDA recommended in August 1994 that the drug be withdrawn from patients except in those cases where the patient's well-being depends on continued use of the drug.

Meanwhile, other new drugs, including vigabatrin, tiagabine, zonisamide, flunarizine, topiramate, and oxcarbazepine, are in, or being considered for, clinical trials in the United States (Table 2). Vigabatrin and oxcarbazepine are now marketed in Europe and zonisamide is available in Japan. This edition will not cover drugs that are not available in the United States.

Although extensive phase 2 and phase 3 testing is performed on all new drugs before FDA approval, this clinical testing of a few thousand patients is not sufficient to exclude rare and idiosyncratic side effects. In the case of felbamate, extensive animal and clinical testing did not suggest any risk for bone marrow suppression. Only after a year of use and prescriptions to more than 100,000 patients did the strong association emerge (approximately 1 in 5,000 patients per year). We cannot now predict what other problems may arise over time with these newer compounds. However, gabapentin and lamotrigine have been used in well over 100,000 patients worldwide and we can only hope that the felbamate experience will not be repeated.

Baseline, CBC, reticulocyte counts, and liver function tests should be done at initiation of treatment with any antiepileptic drug new to the patient. Specific recommendations for follow-up testing have not yet been established.

Gabapentin (Neurontin®, Parke-Davis)

Action and Uses

Gabapentin is a GABA-related amino acid that readily penetrates the blood brain barrier but its specific mechanism of action is not yet clear. Several clinical studies have evaluated the safety and efficacy of gabapentin.[5-6] In a double-blind, parallel design study, 127 patients with refractory partial epilepsy were randomized to placebo or to 1200 mg/day of gabapentin. Twenty-six percent of the treated patients had a re-

Table 2
New Antiepileptic Drugs

Drug	Status in USA	Primarily tested in
Felbamate	approved by FDA July 30, 1993, but aplastic anemia advisory issued August 1994	CP, CP to GTC* Lennox-Gastaut
Gabapentin	approved by FDA Dec. 31, 1993	CP, CP to GTC
Lamotrigine	approved by FDA in 1994	CP, CP to GTC
Oxcarbazepine	USA testing in progress	CP, CP to GTC
Tiagabine	clinical testing in progress	CP, CP to GTC
Topiramate	clinical testing in progress	CP, CP to GTC
Vigabatrin	NDA filed (available in 1996)	CP, CP to GTC
Zonisamide	efficacy studies completed, safety studies pending	CP, CP to GTC Baltic myoclonic epilepsy

*CP=complex partial seizure
GTC=generalized tonic-clonic seizure

duction in seizure frequency greater than 50%, versus 10% of the placebo-treated patients (p=0.042). In the U.S. study, 306 patients with refractory partial epilepsy received doses of 600, 1200, or 1800 mg/day.[6] A dose-related decrease in seizures was observed at the higher doses. In clinical use, doses of 2400 to 4800 mg/day have been used and appear to be well tolerated.

Long-term studies of gabapentin have shown that it is well tolerated and does not lose its efficacy over time.[7,8] More than 100,000 patients have been treated with gabapentin with no major adverse reactions linked to this drug. The FDA approved gabapentin for use in adults as an add-on therapy for partial and secondarily generalized seizures. Its major difference from other antiepileptic medications is its lack of interactions with other drugs. The use of gabapentin in children with epilepsy has been studied.

The age group in which gabapentin may be most useful is the elderly. These patients are most likely to be on many other drugs, and gabapentin may be the best tolerated and least problematic.

Pharmacokinetics

The oral bioavailability of gabapentin is approximately 60% in humans. The time to maximum concentration is 2 to 4 hours after a dose is taken. Gabapentin does not bind to human plasma proteins. After intravenous administration, its terminal elimination half-life is approximately 5 hours.[8,9] The renal clearance of gabapentin equals the total clearance in normal volunteers and is 120 to 130 mL/min. No metabolite has been detected in human beings. After single doses, a linear correlation has been demonstrated between dose and the 2-hour plasma concentration in patients on gabapentin monotherapy.[8,9]

Doses

The initital dose of gabapentin in adults is 900 mg/day in divided doses. It can be rapidly titrated, 300 mg on day one, 300 mg b.i.d. day two, and then 300 mg t.i.d. Doses of 3600 mg/day have been well tolerated in adults, and doses of 4800 mg have been used. Clinical experience has shown that these doses are well tolerated and that doses can be increased every few weeks to the maximal tolerated doses.

Adverse Reactions and Precautions

The most common side effects from gabapentin are mild fatigue and dizziness.[9] Other side effects have been nystagmus, hypotension, diarrhea, muscle weakness, dry mouth, sleep disturbances, slurred speech, decreased alertness, tremor, rash, and nausea. There have been no changes in the hematologic and biochemical parameters.[5]

Gabapentin in very large doses appears to have little toxicity; one patient took 48 g in an attempted suicide. Even though blood levels were inititally over 60 mg/L, renal clearance was rapid and she experienced only minimal symptoms.[10]

Drug Interactions

The major feature of gabapentin is its lack of interaction with other drugs.[10] Unlike the other antiepileptic medications, gabapentin is not metabolized by the liver. It is almost completely eliminated by renal excretion of the parent compound. Thus, it does not affect the concentrations of the other antiepileptic drugs,[11] and may have few interactions with other drugs as well. It may be quite useful in patients who are receiving many other medications, such as the elderly.

Gabapentin:

Neurontin® gelatin capsules, 100, 300, 400 mg.

Lamotrigine (Lamictal®, Glaxo-Wellcome)

Action and Uses

Lamotrigine is a compound that probably exerts its anticonvulsant activity by inhibiting the release of excitatory amino acids. In animal studies it appears that lamotrigine may act at voltage-sensitive sodium channels to stabilize neuronal membranes and inhibit transmitter release, primarily glutamate.[12] Clinical studies have demonstrated lamotrigine to be effective in adults with partial and generalized seizures.[13-16] It was approved for use in December 1994 for adults with complex partial seizures and secondarily generalized seizures. The use of lamotrigine in children with epilepsy has been studied.

Pharmacokinetics

Lamotrigine is rapidly absorbed after oral dosing and is 55% protein bound.[13] Lamotrigine is extensively metabolized and excreted predominantly as a glucuronide. In normal volunteers, the mean terminal elimination half-life is 24 hours. Patients receiving either phenytoin or carbamazepine were found to have a shorter half-life, 15 hours (range 7.8 to 33 hours). In patients receiving valproate, the lamotrigine half-life was 59 hours (range 30 to 89 hours). Serum concentrations of lamotrigine varying from 0.5 to 5 mg/L have been reported after doses of 75 to 250 mg/day in patients.

Doses

Doses of 75 to 600 mg/day have been used in studies of adults with epilepsy. The actual doses used may depend on the tolerance level of each patient. The initial doses of lamotrigine must be adjusted to concomitant medications. If the patient is on enzyme-inducing antiepileptic drugs but not valproate, the dose should be 50 mg/day for 2 weeks, then 100 mg for the next two weeks, and then the dose can be increased by 100 mg each week to a dose of 300 to 500 mg/day. If the patient is on valproate, the initial dose should be 25 mg every other day for two weeks, then 25 mg/day for the next two weeks, then increased by 25 to 50 mg every week or two to a dose of 100 to 150 mg/day.

Adverse Reactions

The most frequently reported side effects of lamotrigine have been diplopia, drowsiness, ataxia, and headache.[14] A higher incidence of skin rash has been observed in patients receiving concomitant valproic acid. No significant changes in vital signs or Cps of concomitant AEDs were noted. SGPT, total protein, folic acid, RBC, hematocrit and hemoglobin did decrease slightly, but significantly.[13] In some studies, doses of lamotrigine have been adjusted to maintain trough serum concentrations between 0.5 to 3.0 mg/L. These concentrations have not produced toxicity.

Drug Interactions

Lamotrigine does not appear to affect the concentrations of other antiepileptic drugs. However, patients receiving valproate have a marked prolongation of lamotrigine half-life, almost double or triple its usual half-life. Thus, lamotrigine must be used cautiously in persons receiving valproate. Patients receiving either phenytoin or carbamazepine were found to have a shorter half-life than volunteers.

Lamotrigine:

Lamictal® tablets, 25, 100, 150, 200 mg.

Felbamate (Felbatol®, Wallace Laboratories)

Actions and Uses

Felbamate appears to increase seizure threshold.[1] Its effectiveness was demonstrated in a number of studies in adults with partial and generalized seizures.[2,3] Felbamate has also been shown to reduce atonic seizures and to improve the global assessment scores in children with Lennox-Gastaut syndrome.[4] In July 1993, the FDA granted approval of felbamate for both add-on therapy and as monotherapy in adults with partial seizures with or without generalization and in children with partial and generalized seizures associated with the Lennox-Gastaut syndrome. As of May 1995, 32 cases of aplastic anemia and 14 cases of hepatitis have been reported to the manufacturer.[17] This represents a rate of aplastic anemia of 1 in 3,000 to 5,000 patients using felbamate. The case fatality rates are estimated to be 20% to 30%, and physicians and patients must read the most current "black box" warning in the package insert before using this drug. Because of its association with aplastic anemia, felbamate should be reserved for those patients for whom there is no other effective alternative treatment. For the time being, it appears that felbamate will be available and likely remain on the market.

Pharmacokinetics

In healthy volunteers, the elimination half-life of felbamate is approximately 15 to 20 hours and the pharmacokinetics appeared to be linear. Time to maximum concentration occurs 1 to 4 hours after a dose is administered. Plasma protein binding is not clinically significant.

Doses

In adults, doses during clinical trials have ranged from 1800 to 4800 mg/day. In children, doses of 15 to 45 mg/kg have been used. With monotherapy, larger doses are tolerated.

Adverse Reactions and Toxicity

Animal studies and clinical trials showed no effect of felbamate on hematologic or hepatic function. No major adverse events were noted during the clinical trials involving more than 2,000 patients. However, after use exceeded 100,000 patients, the high incidence of aplastic anemia and hepatitis became apparent. A number of fatal cases of aplastic anemia and hepatitis linked to use of the drug were reported 1 year after felbamate's approval. Frequent monitoring of laboratory parameters is recommended for those patients needing felbamate for refractory epilepsy. Side effects include insomnia, weight loss, nausea, decreased appetite, dizziness, fatigue, ataxia, and lethargy. There were substantially higher rates of side effects in persons receiving other antiepileptic medications, and conversion to monotherapy often reduced side effects.

Drug Interactions

Felbamate has significant interactions with phenytoin, carbamazepine, and valproate. The concentrations of phenytoin and valproate increase with felbamate. Therefore, when felbamate is initiated, the doses of these other agents should be decreased by 20% to 40% or more. On the other hand, carbamazepine concentrations decrease by about 20%

when felbamate is added to therapy. The concentrations of felbamate are lowered by the concomitant use of other antiepileptic drugs, especially those that induce hepatic enzymes.

Felbamate:

Felbatol® tablets, 400 mg, 600 mg; oral suspension 600 mg/ 5 mL.

References

1. Swinyard EA, Sofia RD, Kupferberg HJ: Comparative anticonvulsant activity and neurotoxicity of felbamate and four prototype antiepileptic drugs in mice and rats. *Epilepsia* 1986;27:27-34.

2. Leppik IE, Dreifuss, FE, Pledger GW, et al: Felbamate for partial seizures: Results of a controlled clinical trial. *Neurology* 1991;41:1785-1789.

3. Sachedo R, Kramer LD, Rosenberg A, et al: Felbamate monotherapy: Controlled trial in patients with partial onset seizures. *Ann Neurol* 1992;32: 386-292.

4. The Felbamate Study Group in Lennox-Gastaut syndrome. Efficacy of felbamate in childhood epileptic encephalopathy (Lennox-Gastaut syndrome). *N Engl J Med* 1993; 328:29-33.

5. Bartoszyk GD, Meyerson N. Reimann W, et al: Gabapentin. In: Meldrum BS, Porter RJ, eds. *New Anticonvulsant Drugs*. London, John Libbey, 1986, pp 147-163.

6. Leiderman DB: Gabapentin as add-on therapy for refractory partial epilepsy: Results of five placebo-controlled trials. *Epilepsia* 1994;35 (suppl 5): S74-S76.

7. Sivenius J, Ylinen A, Kalviainen R, et al: Long-term study with gabapentin in patients with drug-resistant epileptic seizures. *Arch Neurol* 1994; 51(10):1047-1050.

8. The U.S. Gabapentin Study Group: The long-term safety and efficacy of gabapentin (Neurontin) as add-on therapy in drug-resistant partial epilepsy. *Epilepsy Res* 1994; 18(1):67-73.

9. Schmidt D: Potential antiepileptic drugs: Gabapentin. In: Levy R, Mattson R, Meldrum B, et al, eds. *Antiepileptic Drugs*. 3rd ed. New York, Raven Press, 1989, pp 925-935.

10. Fisher JH, Barr AN, Rogers SL, et al: Lack of serious toxicity following gabapentin overdose. *Neurology* 1994;44(5): 982-983.

11. Graves NM, Holmes GB, Leppik IE: Pharmacokinetics of gabapentin in patients treated with phenytoin. *Pharmacotherapy* 1989;9:196.

12. Miller AA, Sawyer DA, Roth B: Lamotrigine. In: Meldrum B, Porter RJ, eds. *New Anticonvulsant Drugs.* London, John Libbey, 1986, pp 165-177.

13. Gram L: Potential antiepileptic drugs: Lamotrigine. In: Levy R, Mattson R, Meldrum B, et al, eds. *Antiepileptic Drugs.* 3rd ed. New York, Raven Press, 1989, pp 947-953.

14. Jawad S, Richens A, Goodwin G, et al: Controlled trial of lamotrigine (Lamictal) for refractory partial seizures. *Epilepsia* 1989;30:356-363.

15. Binnie CD, Beintema CJ, Debets RMC, et al: Seven-day administration of lamotrigine (Lamictal) for refractory partial seizures. *Epilepsia* 1987;1:202-208.

16. Messenheimer J, Ramsey RE, Willmore LJ, et al: Lamotrigine therapy for partial seizures: A multicenter, placebo-controlled, double-blind, cross-over trial. *Epilepsia* 1994;35(1):13-21.

17. Leppik IE, Wolff DL: The place of felbamate in the treatment of epilepsy. *CNS Drugs* 1995;4:294-301.

Chapter 9

Measuring Antiepileptic Drug Concentrations and Patient Compliance

Measurement of antiepileptic drug concentrations is necessary to monitor the treatment of epilepsy. Table 1 lists prudent times to measure the concentrations. A number of devices exists for measuring medication concentrations in plasma, serum, saliva, and other biological samples (Figure 1). Gas liquid chromatography is generally accurate, with coefficients of variation (CV) of less than 5% for standard antiepileptic drugs (AEDs).[1] High-performance liquid chromatography, often used in laboratory settings, has an accuracy comparable with that of gas liquid chromatography.[2] Both methods can measure a number of commonly used AEDs simultaneously. Moreover, inspection of the chromatographic tracing often can point up errors of assay performance. Both chromatographic techniques, however, require highly skilled personnel along with laboratory support systems, and thus have not gained widespread use in clinics.

Table 1
Suggestions for Using Blood Tests in Monitoring Patients with Epilepsy

Antiseizure Medications:*

1. at steady state, good control, and toxicity to get target level
2. to monitor compliance, annually
3. at breakthrough seizure
4. at toxicity

*Trough measurements are primarily useful for pharmacokinetic studies. Levels drawn for target levels and compliance should be obtained at similar times of day, within 1 to 2 hours of each other.

Hematologic/Hepatic:

1. at initiation of therapy
2. once during the first few months
3. whenever clinical symptoms occur
4. annually or less often

Other

1. whenever symptoms occur

In the clinical setting, immunoassays are preferred because they require fewer operator skills. Widely used systems include the Syva EMIT®,

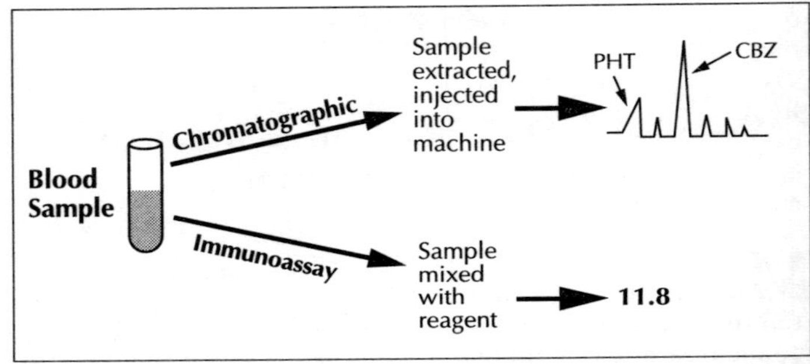

***Figure 1**—Two major kinds of systems are used to measure AED concentrations. The chromatographic system produces a graphic output and measures concentrations as peak heights. Most immunoassay systems have internalized a number of steps, with the concentration determined photometrically after various reactions have taken place. The concentration is usually displayed as a number.*

Abbott TDX®, Ames Seralyzer®, and Syntex Acculevel® systems.[3,4] Other systems are being developed. To be approved by the U.S. Food and Drug Administration, a device for therapeutic drug monitoring must be able to perform with a coefficient of variation (CV) of less than 5%. Although all of these devices meet this standard under strict testing conditions, the potential for error exists in clinical settings. It is reasonable to assume that less than 5% of the variability in serial AED determinations can be attributed to measurement error if testing is done by a certified laboratory. Most of the variability between serial measurements of AED concentrations over time in a patient can be attributed to pharmacokinetics and compliance.

Pharmacokinetics

A number of pharmacokinetic factors can influence the absorption and elimination of AEDs. For example, changes in product formulation can markedly alter the absorption of phenytoin to the degree that toxic reactions can occur.[5] In the case of permissible or mandated generic substitution, product formulations may play a role in creating variable drug concentrations. Alteration of gastric or intestinal absorption by food or other drugs may influence the time or extent of absorption.[6] To a small degree, changes in hepatic or renal blood flow can modify the rate of clearance and affect medication concentrations.[7]

Time of sampling may contribute to variability in AED levels. Phenytoin has a relatively long absorption time (time to maximum concentration of 6 to 12 hours) because of its uptake in the small intestine. Nonlinear kinetics give it an elimination half-life of 18 to 36 hours. Thus, one cycle of absorption and elimination can be on the order of 24 to 46 hours. With more than once-a-day administration, the absorption and elimination phases overlap and the concentration differences are small between peak and trough levels. Carbamazepine and valproate both have shorter absorption times and, during long-term therapy, elimination half-lives of 6 to 14 hours.

Generally, blood samples should be drawn at the same time relative to the dose to be useful for compliance measurements. In a clinic setting, this can be accomplished by always scheduling appointments for the same time of day. Our limit is plus or minus 1 hour. This can be attained most of the time. For example, a person with a 3 PM examination usually has blood drawn by 3:30 PM, but any time between 2:30 PM and 4:30 PM is acceptable.

Compliance

Noncompliance with AEDs is a major factor in the recurrence of seizures in patients

Table 2
Types of Behavior in Noncompliance

Medication Ingestion
- Consistent overcompliance
- Consistent undercompliance
- Irregular
  - irregularly irregular
  - sporadically irregular
  - cyclically irregular

Prescription filling
Medical appointments

Life-style
Sleep patterns
Alcohol use
Psychological stress
Exposure to music, strobe lights
Drug abuse
Adherence to regulations

Intentionality of Compliance
Patient controlled
- Rational
  - pregnant women afraid of teratogenicity
  - compensation-related
- Irrational
  - fear of medicine
  - superstition

Structural
- Memory deficit
- Financial problems

with epilepsy. As many as 50% of all patients with epilepsy are noncompliant to a degree that interferes with optimal treatment.[8,9] Studies using electronic monitors to measure compliance indicate that what may appear to be sporadic seizures can be attributed to missed doses of AEDs.[10] Consequently, proper management of epilepsy requires physicians to identify noncompliant patients, determine the extent of the problem, and devise and monitor an appropriate intervention strategy.

Table 3
Methods By Which Compliance Can Be Measured

Direct
- Measurement of isolated AED levels
- Serial measurement of AED levels to determine variability
- Recording pill-taking behavior with electronic devices

Indirect
- Patient interview
- Therapeutic outcome
- Physician's judgment
- Interviews with caregivers
- Pill counts

AED = antiepileptic drug

The Importance of Compliance

Noncompliant behavior may significantly increase health care costs.[11] An increased number of seizures would result in rising fees for ambulance transportation, emergency department visits, and hospitalization, as well as for medical treatment and drugs. In addition, seizures experienced at work or in recreational settings have social costs. Moreover, noncompliant patients run the risk of endangering others, for example, by having seizures while driving or by injuring an unborn child if seizures occur during pregnancy. Status epilepticus may be associated with subtherapeutic AED concentrations, probably from missed doses.[12]

Treatment of epilepsy requires that stable drug concentrations be maintained at the active receptor site at all times. Unlike pain or infections, for which intermittent attainment of analgesic or bactericidal concentrations is acceptable, epilepsy is best controlled when as little variation as possible occurs over time in medication concentrations. One of the most common precipitants of a seizure is a reduction in drug concentrations, either from missed doses[13] or from an illness that increases metabolism and thereby lowers therapeutic levels.[14]

A patient with epilepsy has a population of hyperexcitable neurons that may generate clinical seizures if modulation of excitatory and inhibitory processes in the central nervous system is not balanced. In addition, only a twofold to threefold difference in AEDs separates the lowest effective concentration from toxic levels. For example, the usual effective range for phenytoin is 10 to 20 mg/L; for carbamazepine, 4 to 12 mg/L; and for valproate, 50 to 100 mg/L. These ranges are much narrower than for most other classes of drugs. Although pharmacokinetic factors can influence medication levels, compliance generally determines whether a stable concentration will be maintained.

Compliance is a multidimensional variable characterized by type of behavior, extent of compliance, and degree of intention (Table 2). Patient compliance with medication ingestion, which most concerns physicians, generally has three patterns: irregular ingestion, sporadic irregularity, and cyclical irregularity. These may well have different causes. Irregular ingestion is most common. Sporadic irregularity may be event related, ie, stemming from a busy week. Cyclical irregularity may be prompted by specific schedules, such as weekend trips.

Some life-style habits can precipitate seizures, such as irregular sleep patterns, alcohol or drug abuse, exposure to psychological stress, or, for photosensitive individuals, exposure to light. Patients may be compliant with a medication regimen but still experience excessive seizures because they are exposed to these risk factors.

Extent of compliance must be viewed as a continuum of behavior, which ranges from the rare patient who takes every prescribed dose precisely as directed, to the consistently noncompliant patient. Most patients fall somewhere between these extremes. Much of the variability in AED concentrations not accounted for by small pharmacokinetically-induced fluctuations can be attributed to noncompliance.

Defining Compliance

There are many ways to assess compliance, but the methods can be divided into two categories: direct or indirect (Table 3). The direct methods involve technologies such as measuring AED levels in blood or using devices that record when patients take their pills. Other studies have used measurements of AED levels in patients' blood to evaluate compliance and identify as noncompliant those whose levels fall outside the usual therapeutic range. Patients whose levels are within normal range are then considered compliant. This method is simplistic, however, because compliant patients may be receiving doses that are too low for their body weight and, consequently, have levels below normal range.

Indirect assessments rely on patient interviews. But interviews and other similar measures, such as compliance ratings by physicians or therapy outcomes, may be inaccurate or biased.[15] However, they are more accurate than suspected.[11]

A patient's compliance pattern may change over time. Fluctuations in medication concentration during times of constant prescribed dose—beyond those expected from assay error or pharmacologic fluctuations—may reflect noncompliance with the prescribed regimen. The degree of fluctuation can be calculated using the coefficient of variation (CV), as described in the equation in Figure 2.

A number of studies have evaluated variability of serial phenytoin and carbamazepine concentrations in various settings. In a study of phenytoin, patients in a residential facility were found to have CV values of less than 10%.[16] In compliant patients in an outpatient study of bioavailability, where samples were obtained every 2 weeks and compliance was monitored by pill counts and interviews, the CV of phenytoin was less than 20%.[16] A few of these patients reported missing an occasional dose several days before the blood sample was taken. This did not significantly affect the CV. In this same study, sequential epilepsy clinic patients were asked about compliance; there was a strong correlation between reported noncompliance and a high CV. Data from rigorous studies indicate that most compliant patients had CV below 20%[17] for carbamazepine. Our experience indicates that similar fluctuations may be expected with valproate.

$$\text{Coefficient of variation (\%)} = \frac{\text{standard deviation} \times 100}{X}$$

X = mean of plasma concentration measurements

***Figure 2**—Calculating the degree of fluctuation by using the coefficient of variation.*

Based on this experience, we have adopted the guideline of the percent deviation from the mean of two or more levels to aid in evaluation of noncompliance. Although calculation of the CV is more accurate, a determination of the percent deviation is simpler and more practical for clinical use. In general, deviation of 20% or less from the mean of previous phenytoin, carbamazepine, or valproate concentrations is evidence for adequate compliant behavior. A patient can attain the 20% limit even if he or she misses an occasional dose (Figure 3). Values between 20% to 45% should raise strong suspicions of noncompliance. Values deviating more than 45% are almost always associated with noncompliance. The larger the percentage, the more marked the noncompliance—assuming the absence of any factors altering the pharmacokinetics, such as new medication, illness, or altered bioavailability. The percent deviation from the mean can be used as a general measure of the degree of noncompliance. For example, a patient with a

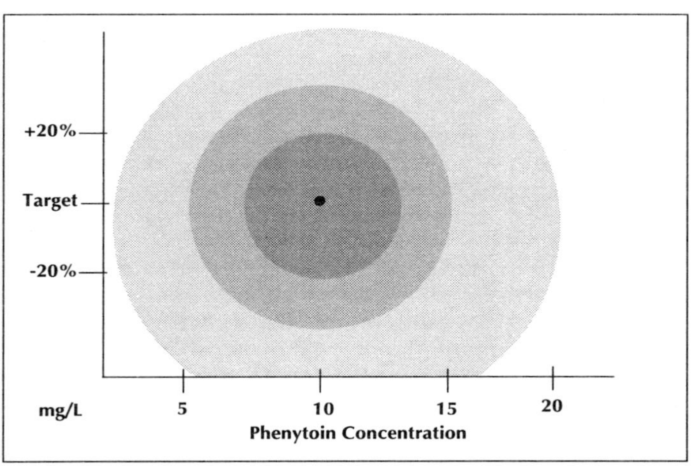

Figure 3*—Representation of allowable variability over time if the target level of phenytoin is 10 mg/L. Levels between 8 and 12 mg/L are within the 20% fluctuation observed in compliant patients. Levels below 5.5 mg/L and above 14.5 mg/L are usually associated with noncompliance.*

Table 4
Examples of Patients From the MINCEP Clinic Illustrating Use of Variability in Serial Levels to Determine Compliance

Pt#	Dates of Visits	Medication	Daily Dose	Level mg/L	
191	8-21-89	PHT	300 mg	26.6	Mean=28.4
	8-23-89	PHT	300 mg	32.4	±20%=5.7
	10-25-89	PHT	300 mg	26.6	Compliant range= 22.7 to 34.4
251	9-28-88	PHT	460 mg	20.8	Mean=23.1
	7-12-89	PHT	460 mg	25.1	±20%=4.6
	1-10-90	PHT	460 mg	23.3	Compliant
	10-24-90	PHT	460 mg	13.1*	range= 18.5 to 27.7
80	2-28-89	CBZ	2000 mg	7.2	Mean=8.6
	5-2-89	CBZ	2000 mg	9.0	±20%=1.8
	10-31-89	CBZ	2000 mg	9.6	Compliant
	2-12-91	CBZ	2000 mg	5.0*	range= 6.5 to 10.4
78	9-27-88	CBZ	1600 mg	9.1	Mean=8.1
	10-29-88	CBZ	1600 mg	7.9	±20%=1.6
	2-21-88	CBZ	1600 mg	6.8	Compliant
	8-22-89	CBZ	1600 mg	8.4	range= 6.5 to 9.7

*Out of range, probable noncompliance
PHT=phenytoin
CBZ=carbamazepine

deviation of ±25% would be less severely noncompliant than one with a deviation of ±35%. A patient with a deviation of ±45% must be considered in need of intervention to improve compliance.

Serial measurements of AED levels are a powerful tool for detecting noncompliance (Table 4). With increasing legal pressure on physicians to certify driving licenses or workplace safety for patients with epilepsy, knowing that a patient is compliant becomes critical. Thus, even if a patient's AED concentrations fall within the usual therapeutic range, but vary from the

Table 5
Strategies to Improve Patient Compliance

Education
- Explain diagnosis and treatment plan
- Discuss the timetable for follow-up
- Provide pamphlets or video presentations
- Arrange for staff to help patient and family understand
- Explain how to implement treatment

Dosing
- Reduce the number of medications
- Reduce the number of doses taken each day
- Provide a dose checklist
- Provide a pill box with a daily compartment or alarm reminder

Clinic Visits
- Increase the frequency of visits
- Designate a specific clinic staff person for contacts

high to the low end, noncompliant behavior must be suspected. That patient may be at increased risk for intermittent toxicity or seizures.

Measurement of serial blood levels is relatively crude compared with the use of a device that records each opening of a medication container daily. Such a device can detect noncompliant behavior lasting only a few days between clinic visits or blood level measurements.[10] However, use of this method is limited now to clinical research because of its cost.

Psychosocial Aspects of Compliance

Another aspect of compliance is intention, which can be patient controlled or structural. Patient noncompliance can be rational or irrational. Rational noncompliance usually arises from a well-defined, logical, and consistent belief system—eg, the pregnant woman who decides to suspend use of AEDs because of concerns about teratogenicity. Although the accuracy of the risk/benefit calculation might be open to question, the decision is founded in logic.

An example of an irrational belief system is one in which a patient believes that seizures are influenced by the moon, and therefore that medications are not needed during certain lunar phases.

Structural reasons for noncompliance are outside a patient's control. For example, a patient who developed epilepsy after trauma to the temporal lobes would have memory dysfunction, leading to difficulty in remembering a medication schedule.

Strategies to Improve Compliance

Some strategies for improving compliance are reviewed by Shope[9] and are listed in Table 5. The most important factor is correctly identifying the underlying cause of noncompliance. Each patient must be considered individually. If the intention toward compliance is being thwarted by external factors, these must be addressed. For example, a patient whose limited financial resources preclude the purchase of expensive medications might be switched to a less costly drug. In contrast, education may be the key if a patient does not understand the short half-lives of AEDs and has not been informed about the importance of taking medication regularly.

References

1. Kupferberg HF: Quantitative estimates of diphenylhydantoin, primidone, and phenobarbital in plasma by gas-liquid chromatography. *Clin Chim Acta* 1970;29:282-288.

2. Wad N: Simultaneous determination of 11 antiepileptic compounds in serum by high-performance liquid chromatography. *J Chromatogr* 1984; 305:127-133.

3. Graves NM, Holmes GB, Leppik IE, et al: Quantitative determination of phenytoin and phenobarbital in capillary blood by Ames Seralyzer. *Epilepsia* 1987;28:713-716.

4. Leppik IE, Oles KS, Sheehan ML, et al: Phenytoin and phenobarbital concentrations in serum: a comparison of Ames Seralyzer with GLC, TDX, and EMIT. *Ther Drug Monit* 1989;1:73-78.

5. Tyrer JH, Eadie MJ, Sutherland JM, et al: Outbreak of anticonvulsant intoxication in an Australian city. *Br Med J* 1970;4:271-273.

6. Dosing M: Effect of acute and chronic exercise on hepatic drug metabolism. *Clin Pharmacokinet* 1985;10:426-431.

7. Levy RH, Unadkat JD: General principles: drug absorption, distribution and elimination. In: Levy RH, Dreifuss FE, Mattson RH, et al, eds. *Antiepileptic Drugs.* 3rd ed. New York, NY, Raven Press, 1989, pp 1-22.

8. Leppik IE, Schmidt D, eds:

Summary of the First International Workshop on Compliance in Epilepsy. *Epilepsy Res* 1988;1(suppl):179-182.

9. Shope J: Intervention to improve compliance with pediatric anticonvulsant therapy. *Patient Couns Health Educ* 1980;21:135-141.

10. Cramer JA, Mattson RH, Prevey ML, et al: How often is medication taken as prescribed? A novel assessment technique. *JAMA* 1989;261: 3273-3277.

11. Green LW, Simons-Morton D: Denial, delay, and disappointment: discovering and overcoming the causes of drug errors and missed appointments. *Epilepsy Res* 1988; 1(suppl):7-22.

12. Cranford RE, Leppik IE, Patrick B: Intravenous phenytoin: clinical and pharmacokinetic aspects. *Neurology* 1978; 28:874-880.

13. Stanaway L, Lambie DG, Johnson RH: Noncompliance with anticonvulsant therapy as a cause for seizures. *N Z Med J* 1985;98:150-152.

14. Leppik IE, Ramani V, Sawchuk RJ, et al: Increased clearance of phenytoin during infectious mononucleosis. *N Engl J Med* 1979;300:481-482.

15. Mushlin AI, Appel FA: Diagnosing potential noncompliance. Physicians' ability in a behavioral dimension of medical care. *Arch Intern Med* 1977; 137:318-321.

16. Leppik IE, Cloyd JC, Sawchuk RJ, et al: Compliance and variability of plasma phenytoin levels in epileptic patients. *Ther Drug Monit* 1979;1: 475-483.

17. Graves NM, Holmes GB, Leppik IE: Compliant populations: variability in serum concentrations. *Epilepsy Res* 1988; 1(suppl):91-99.

Chapter 10

Laboratory Testing

As the public becomes increasingly concerned about the cost of health care, physicians can expect to feel more pressure to cut costs. While facing these pressures, physicians must also consider the overall cost to the patient and to society of not performing necessary laboratory testing. However, the need and cost-effectiveness for routine laboratory testing to detect serious adverse effects to all antiepileptic drugs has come under question.[1,2]

Serious reactions to antiseizure medications are uncommon. Even for felbamate, the rate is less than 1 per 3,000 patients. They include hepatotoxicity, bone marrow suppression, pancreatitis, exfoliative dermatitis, and others, which, if not detected in time, may be fatal. Because of the perceived medico-legal climate, much emphasis has been placed on routine monitoring of hepatic and hematopoietic factors. On the other hand, Canadian medical societies have discouraged the use of routine testing.[1]

The popularity of laboratory monitoring is based on the assumption that subclinical hepatitis or hematopoietic dysfunction can be detected. But elevations of hepatic enzymes of twice the "normal" range are not unusual, and mild leukopenia is a common side effect in patients treated with antiseizure medications. In addition to being costly, laboratory testing may be misleading, provoke further testing, or lead to inappropriate discontinuation of medication.

The cost of performing routine laboratory testing is probably considerable. If one assumes that 2.8 million persons are being treated for epilepsy in the United States, that a set of hematologic and hepatic tests costs $50 (conservatively), and that the test is repeated three times a year for each patient, the cumulative cost would be $420 million. This approximates the annual cost of all antiseizure medication and greatly exceeds the total annual funds being spent on research for epilepsy.

Table 1
Idiosyncratic Reactions to Antiepileptic Medications

Reaction	CBZ	PHT	VPA	FBM	Other AEDs**
	Approximate Rates of Occurrence*				
Aplastic anemia	rate=2/575,000 n=65 (61 adults)	rate=A n=35	rate=A n=1-2	rate=1/3,000 n=32	rate=A n=?
Hepatitis	rate=A n=30	rate=A n=60	see Table 1a	rate=1/10,000 n=14	rate=A n=20
Pancreatitis	rate=A n=a few	rate=A n=a few	rate=A n=10	rate=A n=a few	rate=A n=0
Exfoliative dermatitis	rate=A n=30	rate=A n=30	rate=A n=<5	rate=A n=?	rate=A n=30

A=less than 1/100,000 treated patients
*Data, based on review of literature and hearsay, are incomplete except for hepatitis for CBZ, FBM, and VPA and hematologic disorders for CBZ and FBM.
**Barbiturates and benzodiazepines

Table 1a*
Approximate Rate of Occurrence of Fatal Hepatitis from Valproate

Age	Monotherapy	Polytherapy
infant	1/7,000	1/500
child	1/9,000	1/6,500
adult	0	1/22,000

* Data from Dreifuss et al.[5]

Nevertheless, there are two reasons for the great reluctance in the United States to abandon routine laboratory monitoring. First, there is the perception that on rare occasions such testing may detect a serious adverse event early enough to prevent a fatal outcome. Second, there is the real concern that the medicolegal consequences of not following community practice standards could be very severe. However, support is growing in the literature for abandonment of routine monitoring.[1,3]

Rate of Adverse Effects

The precise frequency of serious drug effects from antiseizure medications is difficult to determine because of inadequate postmarketing surveillance. Most of the information available comes from two sources: reports in the medical literature and information from drug manufacturers supplied to the US Food and Drug Administration.

Tables 1 and 1a list the approximate number of cases of life-threatening reactions attributable to specific antiepileptic medications in the United States, derived from the medical literature. This number is crude, but it underscores the relatively infrequent occurrence of serious reactions. Felbamate is the one exception; its rate for aplastic anemia is approximately 1 in 3,000 to 5,000 treated cases, while its rate for hepatitis is approximately 1 in 10,000 patients.

Carbamazepine was considered to be associated with a high risk of aplastic anemia shortly after its introduction. In a thorough review using estimated number of persons exposed per year,[4] a rate of 2 cases of aplastic anemia for 575,000 treated persons and 1 fatality was calculated. Interestingly, 61 of the 65 reported cases of agranulocytosis or aplastic anemia occurred in adults. Similar data are not available for phenytoin, but such cases have been reported in the literature. Aplastic anemia has rarely been reported in association with valproate, and well-documented cases of aplastic anemia in phenobarbital or other antiepileptic medications are rare. Thus, it would appear that the highest risk group for aplastic anemia is adults exposed to carbamazepine, but this conclusion must be tempered by lack of reliable data for the other medications. Even then, the risk for the highest risk group is very low.

A pattern emerges for the incidence of hepatitis. The highest risk group is infants exposed to valproate in the context of polypharmacy.[5] This may result from the fact that valproate metabolism depends on both cytoplasmic and mitochondrial systems, and the relative production of hepatotoxic metabolites is influenced by the amount of drug passing through each system. The proportion of cytoplasmic and mitochondrial metabolism may be influenced by comedication and changes with age. In addition, the existence of metabolic or neurologic disorders poses a significant risk.[6] The actual number of fatal hepatitis cases attributable to phenytoin is difficult to determine, but the overall number may be approximately 50. Carbamazepine and other medications appear to have a lower rate of occurrence of hepatitis. Thus, the only group at major risk are infants on valproate[7]; adults receiving valproate or other antiseizure

Table 2
Laboratory Parameters: Normal Ranges and Threshold ("Panic") Values for Antiseizure Medications

Hematologic	**Normal Range**	**"Panic" Values**
WBC, total	4,500–10,000/mm^3	below 2.0 mm^3
Neutrophils	1,500–6,700/mm^3	below 1.0 mm^3
Eosinophils	200–500/mm^3	above 600/mm^3 (or 10% or more of WBC)
Platelets	150,000–350,000/mm^3	below 50 mm^3
RBC	3.8 million–5 million/mm^3	below 3200 mm^3
Hemoglobin	11.5–15.0 g/dL	below 10.0 g/dL
Hematocrit	34%–44%	below 28%
Mean RBC volume	83–94 μm^3	above 100 μm^3
Mean RBC Hb	28–32 pg	above 35 pg
Hepatic		
Transaminase (SGOT)	15–40 units/L	above 100 units/L
Transaminase (SGPT)	9–31 units/L	above 100 units/L
LDH	60–200 units/L	above 600 units/L
Alk phosphatase	30–115 units/L	above 300 units/L
γ-glutamyltransferase (GGT)	0–65 units/L	above 800 units/L
Bilirubin, total	0.2–1.2 mg/dL	above 1.5 mg/dL
Other		
Sodium	135–145 mEq/L	below 128 mEq/L
Amylase	may vary	3 x laboratory normal

medications are at very low risk.

Other potentially fatal adverse reactions include pancreatitis, serum sickness reaction, Stevens-Johnson syndrome, and other rare complications. Routine laboratory testing for pancreatitis is unnecessary because clinical symptoms of abdominal pain, anorexia, etc, are dramatic and will lead to specific confirmatory tests. For the others, clinical skills are more diagnostic than laboratory findings.

Problem of False Positives

Table 2 is a list of laboratory tests performed routinely. The "panic" values are those that trigger an immediate response from the laboratory, and may be grounds for considering discontinuation of the drug.

Use of antiseizure medications often leads to values out-

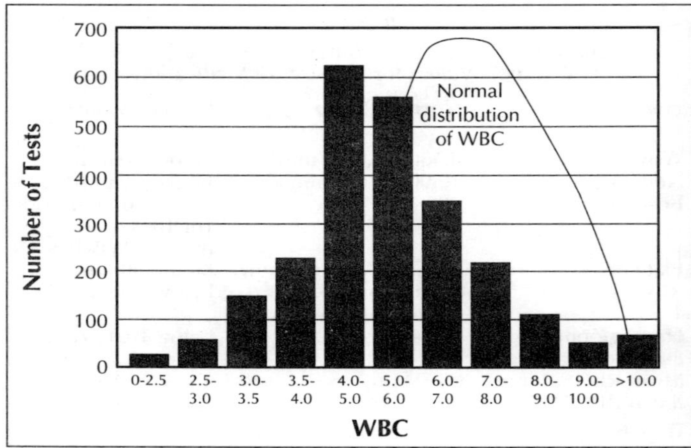

Figure 1*—Histogram of approximately 2,500 WBC values from patients with epilepsy followed at MINCEP over 2 years. Laboratory normal values are from 4.5 to 10.0.*

side of the laboratory normal ranges. A study of 610 persons with epilepsy between 20 and 40 years of age evaluated the effect of long-term treatment on various laboratory parameters.[8] The findings were that leukocyte counts were significantly lower, with a specific lowering of lymphocytes. Also, persistent macrocytosis without anemia was noted. In a reveiw of approximately 2,500 white blood cell (WBC) counts in a population of more than 1,100 patients with epilepsy receiving primarily valproate, phenytoin, and/or carbamazepine, more than 17% had WBC counts below 4,000/cm^3, and eight had a WBC count below 2,500 (1,800 to 2,400)/cm^3.[9] The eight cases with "panic" values were reviewed; all were clinically asymptomatic and, in two cases, the physician discontinued carbamazepine based on laboratory findings. In one patient with AIDS and epilepsy, zidovudine (AZT) was discontinued and the WBC count normalized. In five cases, no change occurred in treatment. The lowest WBC count was 1,800 cm^3. The population with epilepsy had a lower WBC count histogram, but this lowering did not appear to be associated with any clinical problems (Figure 1). Other reports have documented transient leu-

Table 3
1995 Package Insert Recommendations for Monitoring Laboratory Parameters When Using AEDs

Carbamazepine (Basel)	"Complete pretreatment blood counts, including platelets and possibly reticulocytes and serum iron, should be obtained as a baseline. If a patient in the course of treatment exhibits low or decreased white blood cell or platelet counts, the patient should be monitored closely. Baseline and periodic evaluations of liver function, particularly in patients with a history of liver disease, must be performed during treatment with this drug."
Felbamate (Wallace)	"Full hematologic evaluations should be performed before therapy, frequently during therapy, and for a significant period of time after discontinuation of therapy. While it might appear prudent to perform frequent CBCs in patients continuing on this drug, there is no evidence that such monitoring will allow early detection of marrow suppression before aplastic anemia occurs. Complete pretreatment blood counts, including platelets and reticulocytes, should be obtained as a baseline. If any hematologic abnormalities are detected during the course of treatment, immediate consultation with a hematologist is advised."
Gabapentin (Parke-Davis)	"Clinical trials do not indicate that routine monitoring of clinical laboratory parameters is necessary."
Lamotrigine (Glaxo Wellcome)	No specific recommendations.
Phenytoin (Parke-Davis)	No specific recommendations.
Valproate (Abbott)	"Liver function tests should be performed prior to therapy and at frequent intervals thereafter, especially during the first 6 months. However, physicians should not rely totally on serum biochemistry since these tests may not be abnormal in all instances..."

kopenia in up to 12% of adults and children treated with carbamazepine.[10]

γ-glutamyltransferase (GGT) levels are markedly elevated in patients with epilepsy[8] and do not signal hepatic dysfunction. Serum glutamic oxaloacetic transaminase (SGOT, same as aspartate transaminase [AST]) levels may be more reliable. In the MINCEP data base,[9] approximately 33% of values from more than 1,100 patients were above normal; 12 had SGOT (AST) values above 100 IU (normal = 10 to 35). In eight cases, the elevations were sporadic, that is, the values were in the usual range when the test was repeated. In four cases, all on valproate, the medication dose was decreased, and in one it was discontinued. All four had clinical symptoms of loss of appetite, malaise, or nausea, which had alerted the clinician to possible problems that led to testing.

Thus, from the MINCEP data base of more than 5,000 visits, involving more than 1,100 patients who were followed for 24 months, approximately 2,500 WBC and SGOT measurements were obtained.[9] The incidence of WBC counts of less than 2,500/cm^3 was 6.6 per 1,000 patients, and in only two was antiseizure medication therapy changed based on low WBC count.[9] The rate for "panic" SGOT elevations was higher. Nevertheless, clinical symptoms led to tests that uncovered abnormal values. Thus, overall, routine testing alone uncovered only two asymptomatic "panic" values that led to discontinuation of therapy. The approximate total cost of these tests was $125,000. Based on these figures, it is reasonable to conclude that the cost effectiveness of routine laboratory testing is very questionable. This conclusion is aggravated by the fact that most "panic" values were false-positives in the sense that they did not lead to modification of treatment, but only to additional testing.

Camfield et al[3] reported similar results from a smaller series. They performed serial testing at initiation of treatment, at 1, 3, and 6 months, and then every 6 months. There were no serious clinical reactions, but laboratory testing was repeated in 6% of patients to confirm abnormal but clinically insignificant results. In a study of 662 adults in whom treatment was initiated with phenytoin, carbamazepine, phenobarbital, or primidone, no clinically significant abnormalities were detected after 6 months.[11]

Antiepileptic drugs, in addition to the major complications listed in Tables 1 and 1a, can cause other problems that may be associated with clinical symptoms. Valproate may be associated with thrombocytopenia. This in itself may not be problematic if asymptomatic. However, risk of bleeding from injury and surgery may be increased. Carbamazepine is associated with hyponatremia in a substantial number of patients but causes symptoms only occasionally. Elevated ammonia levels may be associated with valproate, but they are probably not significant in the absence of other laboratory signs of liver failure.

Alternatives to Routine Blood Monitoring

Table 3 lists the current recommendations in the product package inserts for monitoring laboratory results of antiepileptic drugs. The present recommendations are less strict than found in previous editions. With the exception of felbamate, none of the other drugs need to be monitored frequently.[12] Screening laboratory testing should be performed to detect any underlying problems before initiating therapy with antiseizure medications. These tests could uncover specific problems that, if they develop further, may be incorrectly attributed to the medication. Rarely, however, do they contradict use of a medication. Table 4 lists recommended tests.

It may be useful to order a CBC check for leukopenia for patients on carbamazepine, or platelets for a patient on valproate 2 to 6 months after onset of treatment. Routine blood monitoring after initiation of therapy is unnecessary if the patient is asymptomatic.

Patients in a high-risk group and those unable to communicate must be monitored more closely. The most efficient moni-

Table 4
Blood Tests to Be Done Before Treatment With Antiseizure Medications

All Patients

CBC, differential, platelets

Serum chemistry (20 channel):

glucose	cholesterol
BUN	bilirubin
electrolytes	alkaline phosphatase
calcium	AST
phosphorus	ALT
magnesium	total protein
creatinine	albumin
urate	globulin

optional: PT, PTT

Specific High-Risk Patients (Based on clinical findings)

Lactate, pyruvate, ABGs

Urine metabolic screen, organic acids

Ammonia

Carnitine

Specific tests for suspected underlying disease

toring system is a high degree of awareness of symptoms that portend serious complications, patient awareness of these, and rapid assessment of any problems that suggest a rare but potentially fatal complication. However, wide acceptance of less routine testing may be tempered by the continued concern about medicolegal liability in the rare but unfortunate case of serious adverse effects.

References

1. Pellock JM, Willmore LJ: A rational guide to routine blood monitoring in patients receiving antiepileptic drugs. *Neurology* 1991;41:961-964.

2. Wyllie E, Wyllie R: Routine laboratory monitoring for serious adverse effects of antiepileptic medications: the controversy. *Epilepsia* 1991;32(suppl 5):S74-S79.

3. Camfield P, Camfield C, Dooley J, et al: Routine screening of blood and urine for severe reactions to anticonvulsant drugs in asymptomatic patients is of doubtful value. *Can Med Assoc J* 1989;140:1303-1305.

4. Seetharam MN, Pellock JM: Risk-benefit assessment of carbamazepine in children. *Drug Saf* 1991;6:148-158.

5. Dreifuss FE, Langer DH, Moline KA, et al: Valproic acid hepatic fatalities. II. U.S. experience since 1984. *Neurology* 1989;39:201-207.

6. Willmore LJ, Triggs WJ, Pellock JM: Valproate toxicity: risk-screening strategies. *Child Neurol* 1991;6:3-6.

7. Scheffner D, Konig S, Rauterberg-Ruland I, et al: Fatal liver failure in 16 children with valproate therapy. *Epilepsia* 1988;29:530-542.

8. Krause KH: Side effects of antiepileptic drugs in long-term treatment. *Klin Wochenschr* 1988;66:601-604.

9. Leppik IE, Jacobs MP, Loewenson RB, et al: Detection of adverse events by routine laboratory testing. *Epilepsia* 1990;31(5):640.

10. Pellock JM: Carbamazepine side effects in children and adults. *Epilepsia* 1987;28 (suppl 3):S64-S70.

11. Mattson RH, Cramer JA, Collins JF, et al: Connective tissue changes, hypersensitivity rash and blood laboratory test changes associated with antiepileptic drug therapy. *Ann Neurol* 1986;20:119-120.

12. Leppik IE, Wolff DL: The place of felbamate in the treatment of epilepsy. *CNS Drugs* 1995;4:294-301.

Chapter 11

Pregnancy and Epilepsy

Approximately 19,000 births occur among women with epilepsy each year in the United States. Clinicians' concerns about caring for women with epilepsy who are pregnant or contemplating pregnancy have raised a number of issues about proper treatment. These include the effect of pregnancy on seizure frequency, the effect of seizures on the fetus, the effect of antiepileptic drugs on the growth and development of the fetus, problems with labor and delivery, the implications for breast-feeding, and the ability of a mother with seizures to care for her child.

The most important aspect in caring for a woman with epilepsy is maintaining an open dialogue between the physician and the patient. Concerns must be discussed before pregnancy, and decisions regarding treatment should consider that conception may occur before the next patient/physician interaction. Although there is a perception that women with epilepsy are at very high risk for adverse outcomes of pregnancy, this presumption is not supported by studies.[1,2]

Seizure Frequency During Pregnancy

In one study of 153 pregnancies in 59 women with epilepsy, seizures increased during 45% of pregnancies, decreased during 5%, and showed no change during 50%.[3] In a review of the literature describing 2,165 pregnancies, 24% were found to experience an increase in seizures, 23% a decrease, and 53% no change.[4] That same study found 12 cases of status epilepticus, the most frightening and potentially serious exacerbation of seizures during pregnancy.[4] In another review of pregnant women with epilepsy, 29 cases of status epilepticus were identified. Nine women died, as did 14 of the fetuses.[5]

Pregnancy is associated with a number of physiologic, endocrinologic, and psychological changes, any or all of which might contribute to lowering the seizure threshold. Women often gain weight during pregnancy, some of which may be caused by increased retention of water and sodium. Some researchers have postulated that these might be responsible for the increase in seizure frequency. However, more recent studies in women with exacerbation of seizures during their menstrual cycles (catamenial epilepsy) have not shown a correlation between seizure frequency, body weight, and total body water.

Plasma progesterone and estradiol levels gradually increase during pregnancy. Chorionic gonadotropin peaks in the first trimester and then drops during the end of the pregnancy. A number of animal models of epilepsy have demonstrated that estrogen has the ability to increase animals' susceptibility to maximal electroshock seizures. Furthermore, focal spikes increase and clinical seizures are exacerbated by intravenous injection of estrogen. However, progesterone may decrease seizure susceptibility in experimental animals and in patients. No comprehensive studies have been done correlating women's endocrinologic changes during pregnancy with alteration in seizure frequency.

The best predictor of seizure frequency during pregnancy appears to be seizure frequency before pregnancy. Almost all patients who had more than one seizure per month in one study had an increase in seizures during pregnancy, whereas women having less than one seizure every 9 months did not experience an increase during pregnancy.[3]

The major factor is poor compliance in taking antiepileptic medication because of fear of malformation in the offspring. In a group of 125 Japanese women, 27% considered to be poorly compliant had a significant increase in seizure frequency during pregnancy.[6] In a study of 136 German women, noncompliance with medication was considered to be a major factor in aggravating seizure frequency during pregnancy.[7]Psychological stress factors, such as anxiety leading to lack of sleep, have been postulated as important in lowering seizure threshold.

Risks to the Offspring

The developing fetus in an epileptic patient is exposed to two sources of risk: the metabolic and mechanical stresses from the generalized tonic-clonic seizures, and the problems caused by antiepileptic medications and their metabolites. As the physician or woman attempts to lower her risks of injuring the fetus by reducing her medication, seizures may occur, which can also harm the fetus. Abrupt discontinuation may precipitate seizures or status epilepticus. Balancing risk from medications against risk from increased seizures requires the exercise of careful judgment based on the most current information.

Effect of Seizures on the Fetus

Intracranial hemorrhage in utero following a maternal seizure has been described in a 28-year-old woman. Since the age of 16 years, she had been treated with phenytoin, 300 mg per day. During the 19th week of gestation she had a generalized seizure. A second seizure occurred in the 28th week of gestation after she missed several doses of medication. After the third seizure, between the 32nd and 33rd week of gestation, the patient felt decreased fetal movement. A sonogram revealed intracerebral hemorrhage with moderate hydrocephalus. There was no evidence of fetal cardiac activity or body motion. Eight days after she had the seizure, labor was induced and the patient delivered a stillborn, macerated male weighing 1,815 g.[8]

Another dramatic report describes a woman who was being monitored during spontaneous labor at term. A spiral electrode had been attached to the fetal scalp for recording the fetal heart rate. Forty-three minutes before delivery, when her cervix was dilated to 6 cm, the patient unexpectedly had a generalized tonic-clonic seizure, lasting 2.5 minutes. Immediately after the seizure, the patient became cyanotic and received 10 mg of diazepam intravenously. Fetal heart rate decelerated to less than 120 beats per minute for more than 13 minutes after the seizure. Twenty-nine minutes after the generalized seizure, late deceleration brachycardia was still observed, and therefore, a cesarean section was performed. Total phenytoin concentration in maternal venous blood was only 0.9 mg/L, suggesting patient noncompliance.[9] Another monitored birth recorded a fetal heart beat of less than 100 after a brief seizure.

These observations indicate that a human fetus clearly becomes asphyctic, as judged by the fetal heart monitoring during and after generalized tonic-clonic seizures. Deceleration in heart rate can persist for some time and has the potential of damaging the infant's development.

While case reports are dramatic, population-based studies give a picture of the extent of the problem. The Collaborative Perinatal Project of the National Institutes of Health found that 4.4 women per 1,000 of approximately 45,000 women had one or more seizures during pregnancy.[10] The rate of stillbirths in women with seizures (not including eclampsia) was 5.14%, significantly higher than the 2.4% in women with epilepsy but no seizures during the pregnancy. Head circumference two standard deviations or more below the mean was significantly greater in women who had a seizure during pregnancy, as was the rate for mixed cerebral palsy and for mental retardation. Thus, it is evident from this large study that seizures occurring during pregnancy can impair fetal development and cause stillbirth.

Complex partial seizures may result in accidents or injuries that may harm the mother, and thus indirectly harm the fetus. An example would be major burns suffered by a pregnant woman as a consequence of a complex partial seizure that required prolonged treatment with a number of drugs. Such a case would subject the fetus to all of the physiologic changes that occur with extensive third-degree burns and to the risks from the multiple drugs used to treat them. Thus, the goal of therapy should be to achieve control of all seizures during pregnancy.

Table 1
Outcomes of Pregnancy From Two Large Population-Based Studies

	Births	Malformations		Relative Risk
Australian Study [1]				
Mothers with diabetes	225	19	(8.4%)*	2.5
Mothers with epilepsy	244	9	(3.7%)	1.1
All other mothers	62,265	2,009	(3.4%)	1.0
Norwegian Study [2]				
Mothers with epilepsy	3,879	170	(4.4%)*	1.25
Control births	3,879	136	(3.5%)	1.0

* statistically significant difference

[2] Used with permission, Bjerkedal T: *Epilepsy, Pregnancy, and the Child.* New York, Raven Press, 1982, pp 289-295.

Fetal Maldevelopment

The risks of malformations in the offspring of women with epilepsy have been a topic of much debate in the literature. Most studies do not clearly delineate the malformations or limit themselves to specific deformities, nor do they review a large enough population with controls. Some population-based studies have shown no significant risk,[1] while others have shown a small but statistically significant risk[2] (Table 1). Smaller studies have shown rates as high as 18.9%.[11]

A recent study that was limited to evaluating congenital heart defects found that of 2,461 live children born to people with epilepsy, the rate of malformation was similar in mothers with epilepsy, in fathers with epilepsy, and in the control population. Thus, the authors concluded that antiepileptic treatment is not a major etiologic factor in congenital heart defects in the offspring of parents with epilepsy.[12] However, other smaller studies have implicated antiepileptic drugs as an etiologic agent for this condition.

The teratogenic potential of phenytoin has been the subject of numerous reports.[13] Animal studies indicate that it has dose-related propensity for causing cleft lip, cleft palate, and cardiac defects. Less common malformations suspected to be associated with phenytoin are bifid ureter and other organ malformations. The types of malformations suspected of being associated with phenytoin, and their relative frequency, do not differ from those occurring spontaneously; thus, the effect of phenytoin may be to increase the rate of spontaneously occurring defects. In one study, the rate of malformations to mothers receiving phenytoin alone was 27.3%,[11] but other studies have reported much lower rates.[14]

A syndrome thought to be specific to phenytoin has been called the fetal hydantoin syndrome.[15] Its features are similar to the fetal alcohol syndrome and consist of major and minor congenital anomalies. The major anomalies include microcephaly, growth retardation, and impaired intellectual functioning. Minor anomalies include strabismus, ptosis, ocular hypertelorism, broad and/or distal phalanges with or without nail hypoplasia, hyperextensible joints, hypotonia, pilonidal sinus, inguinal hernia, umbilical hernia, abnormal dermatoglyphic patterns, and minor club deformities of the feet. These may lead to a characteristic facial appearance. Many of the features seen in the fetal hydantoin syndrome may also be seen with the use of barbiturates.[16] These features have also been observed with all other antiepileptic drugs. The term "fetal antiepileptic drug syndrome" is more appropriate.

Significant neural tube defects associated with valproate have been reported. Data from a registry of spina bifida and anencephaly revealed that these defects occurred in a much higher frequency than expected in children of mothers being treated with valproate.[17] In one study of 12 children born to 11 epileptic mothers, two children were born with microcephaly.[18] Thus, valproate may have a specific teratogenic effect. The risk appears to be 1 or 2 per 100 births, but genetic factors may also play a role.

Carbamazepine also poses a risk for spina bifida. One recent study concluded that carbamazepine has a 0.5% to 1% risk.[19]

Primidone appears to be more teratogenic than phenobarbital by itself.[20] But claims that barbiturates are less teratogenic than other antiepileptic drugs, with the exception of trimethadione, cannot be substantiated by available literature.

Most studies show that the risk of malformations increases with the number of drugs used.[21] Interestingly, the incidence of malformation was the highest (12.7%) in medicated patients who had seizures during pregnancy.[21] Thus the highest risk of fetal injury occurs in women whose seizures are incompletely controlled even with multiple drug use.

There appears to be a strong association between maternal folic acid insufficiency and fetal malformations, spontaneous abortion and placental abruption. A retrospective study examining the effect of folic acid supplementation on congenital malformations from antiepileptic drugs reported that 66 children born to women who received antiepileptic drugs without folic acid had a 15% rate of malformation. These consisted of heart disease, cleft lip and palate, neural tube defects and skeletal abnormalities. A prospective study by the same investigators found that 33 infants born to 22 epileptic women taking folic acid supplements were without congenital malformations and were of normal body weight. Based on these dramatic results a recommendation for folic acid supplementation during pregnancy was made.[22] A study by Dansky[11] supports these results. Use of folic acid supplement during pregnancy is recommended (from 0.8 to 5 mg/day).

A confounding variable is the genetic influence on malformations. One study indicated that children born to fathers with epilepsy had a higher rate of malformations than controls, but other studies are needed to confirm these findings.

It appears, then, that although some studies have reported exceedingly high rates of malformations in women with epilepsy, the weight of the evidence, especially from larger, well-controlled studies, is that the offspring of women with epilepsy have a 1% to 2% risk above baseline of malformations. While some of the increased risk is attributable to antiepileptic drugs, the more likely cause is the complex interaction of genetic factors and environmental factors (drugs, vitamin deficiencies, etc) working in concert. Little data are available regarding human teratogenicity of the newer AEDs. However, animal studies in equivalent species have shown that gabapentin, lamotrigine, and felbamate are not teratogenic.

The American College of Obstetrics and Gynecology has recommended that only phenobarbital, or no antiepileptic drugs at all, be used during pregnancy. This represents an extreme position that fails to consider the many aspects of patient tolerance to phenobarbital, potentially damaging effects on the fetus from that agent, and the problems of switching patients from previously well-tolerated drugs to phenobarbital before pregnancy.

Most of the congenital malformations caused by drugs occur during the first trimester. Therefore, all patients of childbearing potential should be made aware during first contact with their physicians of the teratogenic potential of antiepileptic drugs. How much detail the woman and her physician discuss depends on the woman's plans for the future. Ideally, rational decisions should be made before pregnancy. As a result, the need for antiepileptic drug therapy should be constantly reassessed in women of childbearing potential.

Antiepileptic Drug Pharmacokinetics

Drug absorption. Gastric tone and motility are reduced during pregnancy, resulting in delayed emptying of the stomach. Antacids are frequently prescribed during pregnancy. Dimethicone, a common constituent of antacids, reduces phenytoin absorption by 71%, and kaolin reduces it by 60%, whereas magnesium trisilicate has a negligible effect.[23] Nausea and vomiting are other symptoms during pregnancy that affect drug ingestion and absorption, especially during the first trimester.

Metabolism. Pregnancy prompts changes in almost every aspect of metabolism. A number of changes occur in the liver during pregnancy, and these may affect drug metabolism. The rising concentrations of steroids increase the capacity for hydroxylation, and these substances are competitive inhibitors of microsomal oxidases for drugs such as ethylmorphine or hexobarbitone, and may reduce their elimination.

The fetoplacental unit increases the volume of distribution of drugs that is administered to the mother and also contributes to drug metabolism. At term, the placenta weighs as much as an adult liver and has a blood flow of 500 to 600 mL per minute. The placenta contains the enzyme system for the metabolic pathways: oxidation, reduction, hydrolysis, and conjugation. There are also several forms of cytochrome P-450 in the human placenta. Human fetal tissue is capable of metabolizing numerous drugs at rates that range from 2% to 100% of adult values and significant activity is detectable as early as 6 to 8 weeks of conceptual age. However, such fetal metabolism usually has no clinically discernable effect on maternal drug concentrations because the fetal circulation is so small compared to the maternal circulation.

Protein Binding. Some antiepileptic medications are highly protein bound. Many studies conducted in vitro have shown that pregnancy significantly decreases the plasma protein binding of phenytoin, phenobarbital, valproate, and diazepam.

Specific Antiepileptic Drugs

Phenytoin concentration may decrease dramatically during pregnancy. In carefully studied pregnancies, a change by a factor of 2 in the dose level ratio has been reported. In a prospective study, plasma phenytoin levels were measured during the course of pregnancy in 100 women. Doses were increased when levels fell, and the dose related to level was used to calculate the apparent clearance. Phenytoin clearance increased gradually during the first 32 weeks of pregnancy, reached twice the preconception value during the last 8 weeks, and began to return to normal during the 12-week period after pregnancy.[24]

Phenytoin is a weak acid and is poorly soluble in water. Its pK_a is in the range of 8.3 to 9.2. It is not absorbed in the stomach, but is absorbed in the upper small intestine, and to a lesser degree in the lower small intestine. Very little is absorbed in the cecum or large intestine. Malabsorption may also be related to the use of antacids, which can decrease the amount of phenytoin in solution by forming insoluble complexes.

Phenytoin is highly lipid soluble and rapidly enters the brain. It is stored in the muscle, liver, fat, and other sites that are high in lipid content. It has a rapid redistribution phase and also readily crosses the placental barrier and is distributed to fetal tissues. Pregnancy does not seem to significantly change the volume of distribution of phenytoin.

Any process that increases the mass of P-450 system will increase phenytoin elimination and decrease its half-life. Half-lives of phenytoin during pregnancy have been reported to be decreased by as much as 50%. The fetal liver and placenta are both able to metabolize drugs, which may account for some of the phenytoin eliminated.

Phenytoin is avidly bound by plasma protein. Protein binding is greatly influenced by pregnancy in both humans and experimental animals.[25] In normal women 8 to 15 weeks pregnant, phenytoin binding measured in vitro is within normal limits. However, women progressing beyond the 16th week of gestation have decreased binding of phenytoin to plasma proteins. This change in binding persists for at least 5 days after delivery and returns to normal 5 to 7 weeks postpartum.[26]

These in vitro experiments have been verified by studies of women receiving phenytoin who were followed through pregnancy. This change in protein binding explains in part the observed decrease in total phenytoin concentrations during pregnancy. Nevertheless, this change in binding might not account for most of the documented decrease. Such a decrease, including substantial decreases, could be expected in some unusual situations, especially with the use of comedication such as valproate, which also alters phenytoin protein binding. One study of six women with epilepsy found that the total serum phenytoin concentration was considerably lower the day of delivery. Most of this decrease was explained by a drop in plasma protein binding, but there was a decrease in the unbound concentration, indicating that both increased clearance and binding displacement were responsible. The unbound fraction of phenytoin in pregnant women correlates negatively with serum albumin concentrations[26] and positively with gestational age. Studies of unbound drug concentrations in maternal and fetal blood have shown that for phenytoin the binding in the neonates and the mothers is identical, based on measurements in neonatal cord and maternal blood.[27]

Carbamazepine. Although the decreases in total plasma concentrations are not as great as for phenytoin, carbamazepine levels have been shown in a number of studies to decrease during pregnancy. Evaluation of carbamazepine is complicated by the fact that it is an active metabolite, carbamazepine 10,11 epoxide. As this metabolite has been shown to have antiepileptic effects as well as toxicity and teratogenicity, decisions regarding management of patients on carbamazepine should consider the concentrations of both the parent and the epoxide.

Carbamazepine is absorbed relatively slowly and there is wide variability in its bioavailability. This may stem from its very slow dissolution rate into the gastrointestinal fluid. Alterations of carbamazepine absorption during pregnancy have been demonstrated.

Carbamazepine distributes to lipophilic tissues such as brain and liver. The volume of distribution has been calculated to be 0.8 to 1.6 L/kg. Carbamazepine is rapidly distributed into the fetus. In one study in which eigh pregnant women were given carbamazepine before legal abortion, it was shown that the transplacental penetration of carbamazepine was rapid, occurring over a few hours.[28] It was distributed into fetal liver and kidney, but in contrast to adults the brain concentrations were low in the fetus.

The primary metabolic pathway of carbamazepine is formation of the 10,11 epoxide. In one study of 17 patients on carbamazepine monotherapy during pregnancy, a decrease in concentration was noted throughout pregnancy.[24] This decrease was not as marked as the one observed for phenytoin.

Carbamazepine is approximately 75% protein bound, 25% unbound. No significant change of carbamazepine binding during pregnancy have been reported.

Valproate. Valproate ha been less well studied than other drugs, but decreased concentrations during pregnanc have been noted. In one study the concentration of valproate by the third trimester was found to have fallen to less than one half of the first trimester value

Valproate is available clinically in two basic forms: the acid form, valproic acid, and variou salts, including magnesium and sodium. The acid is very quickly absorbed from the stomach whereas the salts are generally absorbed in the small intestine. Absorption is usually complete because valproate is quite water soluble. There is no evidence that valproate absorption is affected by pregnancy.

Valproate is readily distributed to all tissues. It is present in high concentrations in blood, liver, and kidney and it distributes rapidly to the fetus. It has an apparent volume of distribution ranging from .13 to .23 L/kg in adults.

Valproate is metabolized to a number of compounds, with the two main metabolites being 2-ene and the 3-keto. There is some suggestion that during pregnancy, valproate metabolism may be significantly altered. There is an increased clearance of valproate during the third trimester, which may have multiple mechanisms.

Valproate, like phenytoin, is highly plasma protein bound.[29] Its plasma protein binding is significantly decreased in pregnant women. In one in vitro study, the unbound fraction of the drug was found to be 14.6% in 10 women during late pregnancy, compared to 9.4% in age-matched female controls. Further complicating this phenomenon is the fact that plasma protein binding of valproate is concentration dependent, with the free fraction increasing at higher serum concentrations. Valproate readily crosses the placenta. Concentrations have been found to be higher in the placenta and umbilical cord blood than in maternal serum samples. The fetal/maternal concentration ratio has been reported to be between 1.2 to 3.0, with a mean of 1.7. The neonatal metabolism was measured with a mean half-life of 47 hours, which is much longer than the 8- to 15-hour half-lives observed in adults.

Phenobarbital and Primidone. In almost all studies, phenobarbital concentrations have been reported to be lower during pregnancy. The changes, however, are not as great as those for phenytoin and are approximately the same as for carbamazepine.[24]

Phenobarbital has a pK_a of 7.2 and is readily absorbed from the gastrointestinal tract. Likewise, intravenous and intramuscular preparations are readily absorbed. There has been no evidence that malabsorption of phenobarbital during pregnancy is clinically significant.

Phenobarbital is distributed to all body tissues. It readily crosses the placenta, and concentrations in the fetus and mother have been found to be similar. Unlike most antiepileptic drugs, which are not excreted in the urine, from 20% to

40% of the daily phenobarbital dose is excreted unmetabolized. The degree of excretion depends on the pH of the urine.

Phenobarbital is relatively poorly protein bound compared with other antiepileptic drugs. There is no evidence that changes in protein binding are of any significance during pregnancy. Phenobarbital binding differs between the neonate and the mother. In one study, the unbound fraction was 68% in the neonate compared to 55% in six mothers receiving phenobarbital.

Primidone is metabolized to phenobarbital as well as to phenylethylmalonamide (PEMA). Studies, though small in number, indicate that pregnancy affects primidone metabolism in a fashion similar to that of phenobarbital. Fetal metabolism of phenobarbital has been shown to be present. However, it is doubtful that it exists in a high enough degree to significantly influence the overall serum concentrations in the mother.

Ethosuximide. Ethosuximide is not commonly used during adulthood because it is used primarily to treat absence seizures. In one study of 10 mothers through 13 pregnancies, steady-state serum concentrations of ethosuximide during pregnancy slightly increased, slightly decreased, or remained constant. These effects were variable and small and thus no consistent pattern could be related to pregnancy. Ethosuximide crosses the blood brain barrier rapidly and fetal maternal concentrations are 0.997, indicating that the fetus is exposed to the same concentrations as the mother. Ethosuximide is not protein bound to any significant degree.

Newer Antiepileptic Drugs

Although few studies have been done in pregnant women, we can make several assumptions about the pharmacokinetics of the newer antiepileptic drugs.

Gabapentin is absorbed by an amino acid transport mechanism in the intestine, and pregnancy is unlikely to affect this process. Also, because gabapentin is renally eliminated, and not bound to protein, its concentrations would not be affected by changes in maternal hepatic or fetal placental metabolism or by changes in protein binding.

Lamotrigine absorption may not be affected, but its major elimination pathway is glucuronidation, and studies are needed to determine the effects of pregnancy on its concentrations.

Birth Control

Many studies have shown that doses of oral contraceptives must be increased when women are taking drugs that induce hepatic metabolism of hormones. Of the drugs used to treat epilepsy, the barbiturates, phenytoin, carbamazepine, and valproate, in that order, have the strongest inductive effect. Ethosuximide, gabapentin, and lamotrigine have the least effect.

Labor and Delivery

A frequent problem encountered during labor and delivery is increased tendency for bleeding in the neonate. This can be overcome by the use of vitamin K. The mechanism for this deficit is thought to be the induction of hepatic enzymes by antiepileptic drugs. In general, infant mortality is slightly higher in children born to epileptic mothers than to controls.[5] Vitamin D levels may often be below normal. Interestingly, neonatal jaundice seldom occurs in children exposed to antiepileptic drugs in utero, possibly because of fetal liver enzyme induction. Bone mineralization does not appear to be different in children born to mothers receiving antiepileptic drugs.

Complications of labor and delivery—such as preeclampsia, abruptio placentae, polyhydramnios, assisted delivery, cesarean section, prematurity, and intrauterine growth retardation—may be increased slightly in women with epilepsy.[5]

Drug Treatment During Pregnancy

There is considerable disagreement about the clinical course that should be followed for pregnant epileptic women. Some suggest maintaining stable antiepileptic drug levels throughout pregnancy to prevent seizures from occurring. However, some women do not experience an increase in seizure frequency despite decreased antiepileptic drug levels. On the other hand, some evidence suggests that teratogenicity may be related to drug concentration and that increasing doses could theoretically enhance teratogenicity of the drugs. Perhaps the most prudent course at this time would be to monitor antiepileptic drug levels and increase doses if there is any evidence of increasing seizures. Concentrations of antiepileptic drugs should be measured at least each trimester. Blood should be drawn at each breakthrough seizure to determine whether the threshold has changed (ie, concentrations are as expected) or if there has been a change in clearance or compliance. Sometimes concentrations should be measured more often, such as every few weeks, and the variability between serial measurements can give an estimate of compliance.[30]

Status epilepticus during pregnancy may occur in a woman with epilepsy whose seizures accelerate, or may represent a new onset of seizures in a woman with no history of epilepsy. Loading with phenytoin given intravenously may now be the best treatment available. If given at a rate of no more than 50 mg per minute with monitor, a total dosage of 20 mg/kg can be given safely.[31] Fosphenytoin may replace phenytoin for loading because of its safety. If this is not effective, intravenous phenobarbital in a dose of 10 to 20 mg may be used. Diazepam has too short of a central nervous system half-life to be effective for more than one convulsion. Because status epilepticus in a patient with no history of seizures has a high probability of being caused by a brain lesion such as tumor, arteriovenous malformation, or other condition, MRI scanning should not be delayed until after delivery. A recent study has shown that magnesium sulfate may be a better treatment for seizures associated with eclampsia.[33] However, phenytoin may be needed if longer protection is needed.

Infant Care

Breast-feeding has been an issue of great concern among pregnant epileptic women. Nearly all antiepileptic drugs are transferred in breast milk. The milk concentration to serum concentration for phenytoin is 18%, for phenobarbital 36%, primidone 70%, carbamazepine 41%,[32] and only 4% to 5% for valproate.

The problem of drug effects on breast-feeding is compounded by the fact that half-lives for drugs may be increased in the neonatal period. However, only for phenobarbital and primidone have feeding difficulties and decreased weight gain been definitely correlated with maternal drug ingestion. Conversely, abrupt withdrawal of antiepileptic drugs has been thought to be a factor in isolated cases of neonatal convulsions.

Mothers with seizures can breast-feed and are able to care for their infants. Most problems with child care usually can be attributed to factors other than maternal epilepsy. However, precautions should be taken in some tasks, such as having another person available during bathing of the infant.

Treatment of the Woman With Epilepsy During Childbearing Years

Epileptic women of childbearing potential who wish to avoid pregnancy should be counseled about the possible interactions between oral contraceptives and antiepileptic drugs. Generally, the use of oral contraceptives does not exacerbate seizures, but AEDs that induce hepatic metabolism may diminish the effectiveness of oral contraceptives.

Although women with epilepsy face greater risks than women with no chronic illnesses, these risks are not great enough, with a few exceptions, to preclude pregnancy. The woman and her partner have the responsibility of deciding whether to bear children. The physician's role should focus on providing information about the risks of childbearing and on providing medical care to reduce the risks as much as possible before the patient becomes pregnant. Often overlooked in this are risk factors other than epilepsy that may have much greater consequence on pregnancy than seizures or antiepileptic drugs. These risk factors are, to list a few, advancing maternal age, heavy smoking, substance abuse (alcohol, street drugs), folic acid deficiency, prescription drugs, inadequate prenatal care, and genetic factors.

The most critical step in caring for an epileptic woman of childbearing age is to properly diagnose the syndrome. An accurate diagnosis is essential because a substantial number of women diagnosed as having intractable epilepsy in fact have experienced nonepileptic events (pseudoseizures), and therefore can avoid the risks posed by antiepileptic medications and convulsions.

Antiepileptic medications can be discontinued in some women whose seizures have been well controlled. But attempts to withdraw medications should be made well in advance of contemplated pregnancy. If medications cannot be discontinued, attempts should be made to reduce them to a minimum number and dosage.

Summary

All of the standard AEDs carry some risks, and significant differences in risk of teratogenicity among carbamazepine, phenytoin, and phenobarbital have not been established. The newer AEDs may carry a lower risk. In general, if an antiepileptic drug has been effective before pregnancy and its use has been carefully reviewed, there is no need to

Table 2
Recommendations for Managing Women With Epilepsy Who Wish to Become Pregnant

Before Conception

- Educate the family regarding risks
- Review classification of epilepsy
- Determine most appropriate medicine for seizure control
- Determine need for continued medication
  - may discontinue if seizure-free for 2 or more years
  - do not discontinue medication if epilepsy syndrome suggests continued need for treatment
- Reduce medicines to monotherapy
- Start folic acid
- Eliminate other risk factors—smoking, drugs, alcohol

After Conception

- Do not change antiepileptic medication
- Refer for prenatal care
- Prescribe vitamins, including folic acid
- Check blood levels every trimester and change doses as needed
- Evaluate for neural tube defects at 12 to 16 weeks (ultrasound, alpha-fetoprotein, amniocentesis)
- Consider vitamin K predelivery
- Check antiepileptic drug levels prior to delivery and increase doses if needed

After Delivery

- Check levels
- Examine infant

change to another drug before or during pregnancy. Generalized tonic-clonic seizures occurring during pregnancy appear to be more dangerous to the fetus than the risks posed by antiepileptic drug therapy.

Carbamazepine, phenytoin, and valproate are the most widely used drugs for partial seizures, and no study has demonstrated these drugs to differ in terms of their ability to control seizures. Phenobarbital and primidone appear to have more side effects than most others. Treatment with carbamazepine or phenytoin appears to be the most reasonable course of action once it has been determined that a pregnant woman is at risk for having seizures. For women with idiopathic generalized tonic-clonic seizures in whom valproate has been successful in controlling seizures, changing antiepileptic drugs before or during pregnancy may cause more problems than the relatively small risk of neural tube defects. The other drugs appear to have a similar rate of malformation as valproate, although the types of malformations are different. Furthermore, the other drugs may not control the generalized tonic-clonic seizures as well. Pregnant women on valproate should be warned of the potential for neural tube defects. Although animal studies show that felbamate, gabapentin, and lamotrigene are not associated with significant malformations, human experience is limited.

Whatever the case, quality prenatal care must be provided. Folic acid supplements of 0.8 to 5 mg/day may lower the incidence of malformations.[11] Vitamin K supplementation may be necessary to reduce bleeding problems during labor and delivery.

With optimal care (Table 2), both the patient and physician can expect a favorable outcome of pregnancy in the vast majority of instances. Consequently, epilepsy should not preclude a woman from bearing and rearing children.

References

1. Stanley FJ, Prescott PK, Johnston R, et al: Congenital malformations in infants of mothers with diabetes and epilepsy in Western Australia, 1980-1982. *Med J Aust* 1985; 143: 440-442.

2. Bjerkedal T: Outcome of pregnancy in women with epilepsy, Norway 1967 to 1978: Congenital malformations. In: Janz D, Bossi L, Dam M, et al, eds. *Epilepsy, Pregnancy, and the Child.* New York, Raven Press, 1982, pp 289-295.

3. Knight AH, Rhind EG: Epilepsy and pregnancy: A study of 153 pregnancies in 59 patients. *Epilepsia* 1975;16:99-110.

4. Schmidt D: The effect of pregnancy on the natural history of epilepsy: Review of the literature. In: Janz D, Bossi L, Dam M, et al, eds. *Epilepsy, Pregnancy, and the Child.* New York, Raven Press, 1982, pp 3-14.

5. Teramo K, Hiilesmaa VK: Pregnancy and fetal complications in epileptic pregnancies: Review of the literature. In: Janz D, Bossi L, Dam M, et al, eds. *Epilepsy, Pregnancy, and the Child.* New York, Raven Press, 1982, pp 53-59.

6. Otani K: Risk factors for the increased seizure frequency during pregnancy and puerperium. *Folia Psychiatr Neurol Jpn* 1985;39(1):33-41.

7. Schmidt D, Canger R, Avanzini G, et al: Change of seizure frequency in pregnant epileptic women. *J Neurol Neurosurg Psychiatry* 1983;46 (8):751-755.

8. Minkoff H, Schaffer RM, Delke I, et al: Diagnosis of intracranial hemorrhage in utero after a maternal seizure. *Obstet Gynecol* 1985;22S-24S.

9. Teramo K, Hiilesmaa VK, Bardy A, et al: Fetal heart rate during a maternal grand mal epileptic seizure. *J Perinat Med* 1979;7:3-6.

10. Nelson KB, Ellenberg JH: Maternal seizure disorder, outcome of pregnancy, and neurologic abnormalities in children. *Neurology* 1982;32(11): 1247-1254.

11. Dansky L, Andermann E, Rosenblatt D, et al: Anticonvulsants, folate levels, and pregnancy outcome: a prospective study. *Ann Neurol* 1987;21:176-182.

12. Friis ML, Hauge M: Congenital heart defects in liveborn children of epileptic patients. *Arch Neurol* 1985;42:374-376.

13. Yerby MS, Leppik IE: Epilepsy and the outcomes of pregnancy. *J Epilepsy* 1990;3: 193-199.

14. Granstrom ML, Hiilesmaa VK: Malformations and minor anomalies in the children of epileptic mothers: preliminary results of prospective Helsinki study. In: Janz D, Bossi L, Dam M, et al, eds. *Epilepsy, Pregnancy and the Child.* New York, Raven Press, 1982, pp 303-307.

15. Hanson JW, Myrianthopoulos NC, Sedgwick-Harvey MA, et al: Risks of the offspring of women treated with hydantoin anticonvulsants with emphasis on the fetal hydantoin syndrome. *J Pediatr* 1976;89:662-668.

16. Seip M: Growth retardation dysmorphic facies and minor malformations following massive exposure to phenobarbital in utero. *Acta Paediatr Scand* 1976;65:617-621.

17. Robert E, Giubaud P: Maternal valproic acid and congenital neural tube defects. *Lancet* 1982;2:937.

18. Robert E, Robert JM, Lapras C: L'acide valproique est-il teratogene? *Rev Neurol* 1983;139:445-447.

19. Rosa FW: Spina bifida infants of women treated with carbamazepine during pregnancy. *N Engl J Med* 1991;324: 674-677.

20. Myhre SA, Williams R: Ter-

atogenic effects associated with maternal primidone therapy. *J Pediatr* 1981;99(1): 160-162.

21. Nakane Y, Okuma T, Takahaski R, et al: Multi-institutional study of the teratogenicity and fetal toxicity of antiepileptic drugs: a report of a collaborative study group in Japan. *Epilepsia* 1980;21(6): 663-680.

22. Biale Y, Lewenthal H: Effect of folic acid supplementation on congenital malformations due to anticonvulsant drugs. *Eur J Obstet Gynecol Reprod Biol* 1984;18:211-216.

23. McElnay JC: Interaction of phenytoin with antacid constituents and kaolin. *Br J Pharmacol* 1981;70:126-127.

24. Bardy AH, Teramo K, Hiilesmaa VK: Apparent plasma clearances of phenytoin, phenobarbital, primidone, and carbamazepine during pregnancy: results of a prospective Helsinki study. In: Janz D, Bossi L, Dam M, et al, eds. *Epilepsy, Pregnancy and the Child.* New York, Raven Press, 1982, pp 141-145.

25. Stock B, Dean M, Levy G: Serum protein binding of drugs during and after pregnancy in rats. *J Pharmacol Exp Ther* 1979;212(2):264-268.

26. Dean M, Stock B, Patterson RJ, et al: Serum protein binding of drugs during and after pregnancy in humans. *Clin Pharmacol Ther* 1980;28:253-261.

27. Friel P, Yerby M, McCormick K: Use of unbound drug concentrations to determine neonatal anticonvulsant exposure. *Epilepsy Res* 1987;1:70-73.

28. Pynnonen S, Kanto J, Sillanpaa M, et al: Carbamazepine: placental transport, tissue concentrations in fetus and newborn, and level of milk. *Acta Pharmacol Toxicol* 1977;41:244-253.

29. Riva R, Albani F, Contin M, et al: Mechanism of altered drug binding to serum proteins in pregnant women: studies with valproic acid. *Ther Drug Monit* 1984;6:25-30.

30. Leppik IE, Cloyd JC, Sawchuk RJ, et al: Compliance and variability of plasma phenytoin levels in epileptic patients. *Ther Drug Monit* 1979; 1:475-483.

31. Leppik IE: Status epilepticus. *Neurol Clin* 1986;4(3):633-643.

32. Kaneko S, Suzuki K, Sato T, et al: The problems of antiepileptic medication in the neonatal period: Is breastfeeding advisable? In: Janz D, Bossi L, Dam M, et al, eds. *Epilepsy, Pregnancy, and the Child.* New York, Raven Press, 1982, pp 343-348.

33. Lucas MJ, Leveno KJ, Cunningham FC: A comparison of magnesium sulfate with phenytoin for the prevention of eclampsia. *N Engl J Med* 1995; 333:201-205.

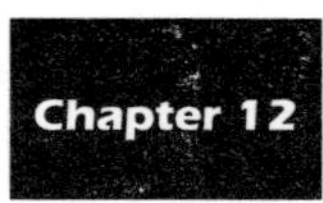

Status Epilepticus

Status epilepticus (SE) is defined as a condition characterized by an epileptic seizure that is so frequently repeated or so prolonged as to create a fixed and lasting condition.[1] SE is a medical emergency that requires prompt and appropriate treatment. Any type of epileptic seizure can develop into SE. The syndrome most commonly associated with SE is tonic-clonic (convulsive) status epilepticus; an estimated 60,000 to 150,000 persons in the United States will have at least one episode of convulsive SE in a given year.

In convulsive SE, the patient suffers from repeated generalized tonic-clonic (GTC) seizures without recovering consciousness and remains in the postictal state between seizures. GTC seizures usually last for 2 to 3 minutes, during which the patient convulses violently. Because of the tonic axial muscle contraction, respiration is halted. During the clonic phase, small amounts of air may be exchanged. The patient often appears cyanotic because of desaturation of the hemoglobin and because of increased intrathoracic pressure impeding venous return. Immediately after the GTC seizure, respiratory drive increases and the patient has deep, rapid respiration. If the SE is not caused by an acute central nervous system (CNS) insult, the level of consciousness may increase before the next seizure; but if there is no improvement in consciousness, a new CNS insult should be suspected (Table 1, Group II).

In adults, GTC seizures are usually followed by 20 to 30 minutes of the postictal state, which is then followed by another seizure. In children, GTC seizures may be continuous. Repeated GTC seizures can lead to systemic cardiovascular dysfunction. The cardiovascular system is particularly stressed from the excessive demands placed on it by the repeated tonic contractions of the skeletal muscle system. Tachycardia is inevitable; bradycardia may occur from vagal tone modulated by CNS

Table 1
Static or Acute CNS Pathology as Causes of Status Epilepticus*

Group I - Static

- Exacerbation of seizures in patients with epilepsy
- Alcohol or drug abuse
- Withdrawal from drugs
- Miscellaneous or undetermined (no acute CNS lesion or metabolic cause identified)

Group II - Acute

- Anoxic encephalopathy
- Acute vascular event (stroke, intercerebral hemorrhage)
- CNS neoplasm
- Acute trauma
- Metabolic encephalopathy
- Meningitis

* Modified from Cranford et al[3]

activity; and cardiac arrhythmias may occur from hyperkalemia. Drugs used to treat SE may contribute to these problems; barbiturates may depress the myocardium, and phenytoin and its solvent, propylene glycol, may cause arrhythmias and hypotension.

While a single GTC seizure is usually followed by great respiratory effort stimulated by hypercarbia, respiratory failure may occur after a series of seizures. The disorder that precipitates SE can itself depress respiratory drive, as can barbiturates and benzodiazepines used to treat the patient. Altered lymph flow may induce pulmonary edema. Rhabdomyolysis leads to myoglobinuria and may cause renal failure. The metabolic-biochemical complications of GTC seizures include respiratory and metabolic acidosis, anoxemia, hyperazotemia, hyperkalemia, hypoglycemia, and hyponatremia. Massive activation of both sympathetic and parasympathetic systems leads to severe autonomic nervous system disturbances, including hyperpyrexia, excessive sweating, and salivary and tracheobronchial hypersecretion. Endocrine abnormalities—including marked elevations in plasma prolactin, in glucagon, in growth hormone, and in adrenocorticotrophic hormone (ACTH)—have been reported. There may also be cerebrospinal fluid pleocytosis attributable to SE.

Mortality and Morbidity

Damage to the CNS may be caused by the systemic effects of the seizures described above or by prolonged electrical discharges within the brain. Prolonged electrical activity within the CNS may cause irreversible neuronal damage. Meldrum and coworkers have shown in animal models that if the abnormal electrical activity is not suppressed, neuronal damage results even when animals are paralyzed and ventilated to prevent the metabolic consequences of the convulsions.[2] Animal brains appear to have a tolerance to 30 to 60 minutes of continuous electrical activity; but after 60 minutes, irreversible nerve cell damage and death are evident. The developing brain is also vulnerable to seizure activity, and permanent damage can occur in the neonatal brain.

What Causes Status Epilepticus?

The reported causes of convulsive SE vary and reflect the population served by hospitals. Two broad groups of patients can be identified (Table 1): those with no new structural CNS lesion (Group I) and those with an acute CNS injury (Group II). Group I includes patients with a history of epilepsy who have an acute exacerbation of seizures. Withdrawal from antiepileptic drugs causes exacerbation of seizures in most of these patients and may be documented by measuring drug serum levels. Drug abuse involving crack cocaine, amphetamines, phencyclidine (PCP, "angel dust") or other street drugs may trigger SE. Unusual causes for seizure exacerbation include baclofen withdrawal or secondary hyperparathyroidism. Prognosis for Group I patients is generally good if treatment is instituted quickly.

Group II patients are those with an acute neurologic insult, such as head injury, rapidly growing brain tumor, anoxic encephalopathy, meningitis, encephalitis, or other acute CNS process. Prognosis for Group II patients is usually poor. They often have seizures after phenytoin loading and often need phenobarbital loading. If this is ineffective, they may need phenobarbital coma. Mortality rates may be as high as 33%,[3] but in most cases, mortality can be attributed to the condition that caused the Group II SE, ie, anoxic encephalopathy.

Not all patients appearing to have continuous seizures are

having convulsive status epilepticus. The syndrome of nonepileptic SE, in which a person has serial nonepileptic convulsions (pseudoseizures), must be considered whenever there is an unusual presentation for the seizure type or if response to antiepileptic drugs does not follow the expected pattern. Occasionally, a person with intermittent decorticate or decerebrate posturing may be mistakenly diagnosed as having SE.

Treatment

Time is critical in the appropriate treatment of SE. Every facility likely to treat SE should have a sequence of treatment to be instituted because it is easy for clinicians to be distracted by other pressing needs.

Figure 1 and Table 2 reflect the protocol developed for use in our facility. The first few minutes should be spent assessing the patient's overall condition. An examination should be made for clues that might indicate an etiology for the particular episode of SE. Medical alert bracelets worn by persons with epilepsy may provide helpful information. Evidence of a recent head injury may suggest the presence of an intracere-

Table 2
Time Frame for Treatment of Status Epilepticus

0-9 min	Assess cardiorespiratory function, obtain history, and perform neurologic and physical examination. Test blood for antiepileptic drug levels, glucose, BUN, electrolytes, metabolic screen, and drug screen. Insert oral airway and administer oxygen if needed. Start IV infusion with saline solution. Administer 25 g of glucose and B vitamins.
10-40 min	Begin infusion of phenytoin (or fosphenytoin), 20 mg/kg, at a rate no faster than 50 mg/min. This may take 20-40 minutes. Monitor EKG and blood pressure. Lorazepam (4 to 8 mg) or diazepam (10 to 20 mg) may be given if convulsions occur while phenytoin is being infused.
If seizures persist	Give phenobarbital, 10 mg/kg at 100 mg/min intravenously. Be prepared to intubate.
If seizures persist	Initiate pentobarbital coma or general anesthesia using agents with which the facility is familiar.

bral hematoma. Historical details surrounding the onset of SE should be obtained. Such information can often be provided by paramedical personnel or by friends or relatives accompanying the patient. Diagnostic laboratory testing should be done to rule out metabolic causes of seizures. SE from hypoglycemia, hyponatremia, and other metabolic conditions do not respond to antiepileptic medications. Drug therapy should begin as soon as it becomes clear that the patient meets the criteria for treatment. The most important clinical sign is recovery of consciousness. This is why we use benzodiazepines sparingly and only if the onset of another convulsion is heralded by low-amplitude clonic activity.

The ideal drug for the treatment of SE should: be administered quickly; enter the brain rapidly; have an immediate anticonvulsant effect; not depress consciousness or respiratory function; have a long half-life (many hours); and effectively block both the somatic manifestations of seizures and the neuronal discharges. No available drug meets all of these criteria; the benzodiazepines act quickly but are CNS depressants with short-action

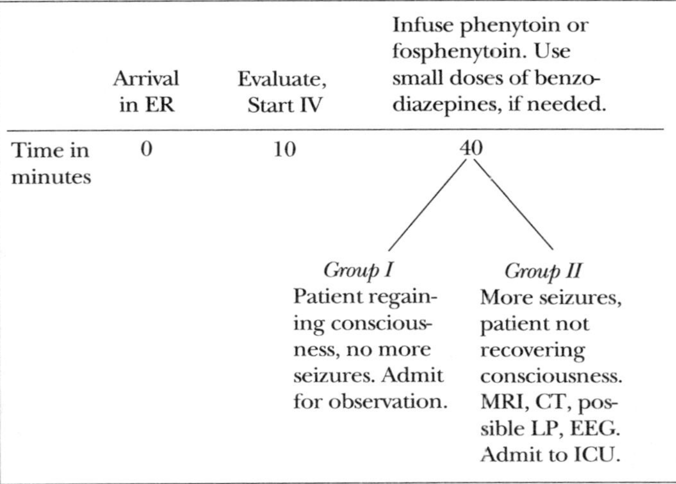

Figure 1—*Time frame for the treatment of status epilepticus.*

times. Phenytoin is long-acting but must be given slowly.

Diazepam

Diazepam became popular in the mid-1960s after a few case reports indicated its success in treating SE. Its profile of activity is a function of the drug's physiochemical properties. Because approximately 20% of cardiac output goes to the brain, as much as 20% of an intravenous dose of diazepam enters the CNS after injection, accounting for the rapid onset of anticonvulsant activity of this drug.

However, the binding of diazepam to the benzodiazepam receptor site is relatively weak. Furthermore, diazepam is also quite lipid soluble and, with recirculation, the relatively high initial brain concentrations decrease quickly as diazepam is redistributed to the greater bulk of fatty tissue. Thus, the duration of diazepam's effectiveness in the brain is less than 30 minutes. Its short, cerebral half-life has been demonstrated in cat models through simultaneous measurements of EEG recordings and of blood and brain concentrations.[4] A similar time course has been observed in the treatment of clinical SE when a significant number of patients receiving diazepam alone had recurrence of seizures.[3] In view of these findings, it is no longer sufficient simply to administer a dose of diazepam, return to other pressing duties, and plan for additional treatment only if seizures reoccur. Instead, diazepam should be used in conjunction with, or be followed by, loading with a medication with a longer course of action in the CNS.

Lorazepam

Lorazepam has higher affinity binding to the benzodiazepam receptor sites when compared to diazepam, and, theoretically, a longer effective life at the receptor site.

In the first double-blind, random study of benzodiazepines in SE (N = 78), a single 4-mg dose of lorazepam was compared with a 10-mg dose of diazepam and found to be equivalent in terms of effectiveness and number of side effects.[5] Overall, one or two consecutive doses of diazepam (10 mg) or lorazepam (4 mg) were effective in 76% and 89% of 81 episodes, respectively. Depression of respiration in some patients was observed with both medications (Table 3).

Because this study[5] was double-blind and many of the subjects would receive diazepam, the protocol's safety component required that all patients be given an 18 mg/kg phenytoin load 0.5 hour after the infusion of the study drug, regardless of whether seizures had occurred. Therefore, this trial could not answer the question of differences in the duration of action of the two study drugs.

At this time, lorazepam has been approved in Canada for use in SE; approval in the United States for use in SE is pending. Clonazepam has been used successfully in Europe for the treatment of SE, but a parenteral form is not available in the United States.

The role of benzodiazepines in SE is limited because they depress consciousness and respiration. These adverse effects may be critical during assessment of the level of consciousness after a series of seizures. Return of consciousness after GTC seizure is typical of a Group I patient, while no

Table 3

Adverse Event Data From 81 Episodes of Status Epilepticus in 78 Patients From a Double-Blind Study of Diazepam vs Lorazepam[5]

Number of patients with adverse events	Patient age (yrs)	Dose (mg)	Adverse event	Severity	Associated diagnoses
Diazepam					
12% (5/41)	55	15	Respiratory arrest	+++	0
	96	10	Respiratory arrest	+	0
	32	10	Sedation	++	0
	64	10	Respiratory depression	++	0
	50	10	Respiratory depression	+	0
Lorazepam					
12% (5/40)	54	4	Respiratory depression	+++	1
	69	4	Respiratory depression	++	2
	57	4	Respiratory arrest	+++	3
	86	4	Respiratory arrest	++	4
	71	4	Hypotension	++	0

+=Mild ++=Moderate +++=Severe

0=None 1=Diabetes mellitus, sepsis 2=Alcoholism

3=Active gastrointestinal bleeding

4=Renal failure, pneumonia, cardiac disease

change or deepening of stupor or coma after a seizure may alert the physician that this is a Group II patient (Figure 1). In addition, since benzodiazepines depress respiratory drive, postictal monitoring of respiration is crucial after using this class of drug; the physician should therefore be ready to intubate if necessary.

Phenytoin

The main advantages of phenytoin are its effectiveness in controlling convulsions, its relatively long half-life, and its lack of significant CNS depression. Its disadvantages include cardiovascular toxicity when given too rapidly, the time required for administering the full loading dose, its relative ineffectiveness in suppressing focal epileptic activity, and venous sclerosis or skin necrosis at injection site. Phenytoin is effective in suppressing experimental seizures as soon as adequate brain concentrations are attained, which, in rats, is within a few minutes.[6] In humans, high brain concentrations of phenytoin are achieved within 30 minutes.[7]

The available preparation of phenytoin contains propylene glycol and ethanol, and it may be diluted to 5 mg/mL or less in normal saline solution to permit steady administration by infusion equipment using an IV filter.[8] Injection of a bolus of undiluted phenytoin by hand can be dangerous if given too rapidly. Both blood pressure and electrocardiographic (ECG) tracings should be monitored during phenytoin infusion. In some situations (eg, tricyclic antidepressant overdose, in which hypotension can be a cardinal feature of SE) the use of phenytoin needs to be monitored closely. In the intensive care unit, the administration of phenytoin to a critically ill patient may be associated with more hypotension and/or cardiac abnormalities. Fosphenytoin is a much safer preparation and should be used instead of phenytoin when it becomes available.

The addition of barbiturates can depress myocardial contractility and decrease blood pressure even further. If the seizures do not respond to phenytoin infusion, there is a high probability that a significant acute CNS insult has occurred and that the patient belongs to Group II.

After a dose of 18 mg/kg, most patients attain serum concentrations between 25 and 30 mg/L (Figure 2).

The volume of distribution of phenytoin in adults is 0.78 L/kg.[9] This means that a loading dose of 20 mg/kg will result in blood concentration of approximately 26 g/mL at the end of infusion (assuming the level was zero prior to the load). Depending on the patient's metabolism, these concentrations are maintained between 15 and 20 mg/L over 24 hours, and additional phenytoin need not be given. The patient's weight can be estimated, and most clinicians can guess the weight to within 15%. The half-life of phenytoin after doses of 18 to 20 mg/kg is in excess of 36 hours.[9] Thus, after one load of phenytoin, blood levels will remain high for many hours. Brain concentrations of phenytoin in humans parallel blood concentrations after 30 minutes.[7] If seizures continue after a loading dose of phenytoin, other agents should be used because the administration of more phenytoin will result in toxic levels and in possibly precipitating more seizures. The kinetics of intravenous phenytoin have not been well studied in children, but it would be expected that the volume of distribution and thus the loading dose would be similar to that in adults.

To make phenytoin more water soluble and avoid the risks of the standard IV prepa-

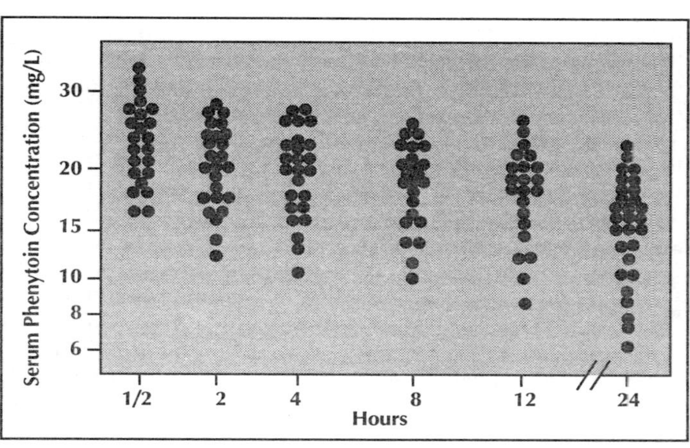

Figure 2—Serum concentrations after doses of 18 mg/kg. The patient's weight was estimated, accounting for some of the scatter. Preloading concentrations were obtained, and any patient with measurable phenytoin concentrations was excluded. Data from Cranford et al.[9] Used with permission, Neurology *1978.*

Table 4
Treatment Protocol for Status Epilepticus With Pentobarbital Coma

Setting
- ICU
- Intubation
- EEG monitoring

Loading
- 5 mg/kg IV over 2 to 3 minutes

Maintenance
- 5 mg/kg/hr

Drug Levels
- 24 to 45 mg/L

rations, a phosphate group has been added to phenytoin (fosphenytoin). Phosphorylases cleave the phosphate, generating phenytoin in the body. This conversion is complete 15 to 30 minutes after administration. This preparation is very water soluble, well tolerated, and, unlike phenytoin, can be given IM.[10]

Phenobarbital

Phenobarbital has the advantages of a long half-life and effectiveness in both generalized and partial seizures. It can also be administered more rapidly than phenytoin. Phenobarbital's disadvantages are that it depresses consciousness and respiration; the respiratory depression may be more profound in a patient initially treated with diazepam. Phenobarbital's volume of distribution is approximately 1, meaning that 1 mg/kg should result in a serum concentration of approximately 1 g/mL. A loading dose of approximately 10 mg/kg of phenobarbital is often used and can be followed by an additional dose of 10 mg/kg if needed. When a patient has been given a load of phenobarbital, an EEG must be obtained because the brain may continue to have electrical seizure activity in the absence of visible motor seizures. Also, patients not recovering consciousness after convulsions may be having "subtle status epilepticus" and need further treatment.[12]

Pentobarbital Coma

If a patient continues to have SE, either with only electrical discharges in the EEG or with continued motor seizures, pentobarbital coma should be instituted. This should be done in an intensive care unit (ICU) and should involve a neurologist and an anesthesiologist.

Pentobarbital coma has been successfully used in SE refractory to diazepam, phenytoin or other drugs.[11] Its use needs to be carefully monitored by EEG recording. Doses should be tailored to maintain a burst suppression pattern on the EEG (Figure 2). Treatment with pentobarbital coma may be required for many days or even weeks. Table 4 provides a protocol for pentobarbital coma.

Treatment of SE in Infants and in Children

Diagnosis of SE in the neonate may be difficult because the seizures are subtle, with symptoms including sucking, random eye movements, stretching, yawning, bicycling movements of the legs, and apnea.[13] Seizures in neonates are unlike those seen in older persons because of the lack of myelin and dendritic connections. Nevertheless, these seizures are often associated with serious CNS disturbances. A standard loading dose of 20 to 25 mg/kg of phenobarbital has been found to be effective.[14] This may be followed by a dose of phenytoin, 20 mg/kg. In addition to these drugs, benzodiazepines are used by some pediatricians. Paraldehyde is useful in some instances; however, its availability is becoming limited in the United States and it may become unavailable in the future.

Nonconvulsive generalized SE consists of frequent or continuous absence seizures and is characterized clinically by clouding of consciousness. The EEG usually shows typical 3-Hz, generalized spike-and-wave discharges. Although absence status is most common in children and adolescents, it is occasionally reported in adults. Complex partial SE may present with clinical behavior ranging from a "twilight" state, with partial responsiveness and semipurposeful automatisms, to total unresponsiveness, speech arrest, and stereotypical automatisms. Aphasic SE, characterized by episodes of inability to speak that last from a few hours to several days, must be considered in patients presenting with dysphasia or aphasia with no other findings of cerebrovascular disease. Fortunately, the EEG is usually diagnostic for these conditions; treatment with benzodiazepam (during the EEG) often results in a rapid normalization of the EEG and clearing of the sensorium. The differential diagnosis of an acute confusional state should always include absence ("petit mal") SE and complex partial SE.

References

1. Gastaut H: Clinical and electroencephalographic classification of epileptic seizures. *Epilepsia* 1970;11:102-113.

2. Meldrum B: Psychological changes during prolonged seizures and epileptic brain damage. *Neuropediatrics* 1978;9:203-212.

3. Cranford RE, Leppik IE, Patrick B, et al: Intravenous phenytoin in acute treatment of seizures. *Neurology* 1979;29: 1474-1479.

4. Celesia GG, Booker HE, Sato S: Brain and serum concentrations of diazepam in experimental epilepsy. *Epilepsia* 1974;15:417-425.

5. Leppik IE, Derivan AT, Homan RW, et al: Double-blind study of lorazepam and diazepam in status epilepticus. *JAMA* 1983;249(11):1452-1454.

6. Leppik IE, Sherwin AL: Intravenous phenytoin and phenobarbital: anticonvulsant action, brain content, and plasma binding in rat. *Epilepsia* 1979;20:201-217.

7. Wilder BJ, Ramsay E, Wilmore LJ, et al: Efficacy in intravenous phenytoin in the treatment of status epilepticus. *Ann Neurol* 1977;1:511-518.

8. Cloyd JC, Bosch DE, Sawchuk RJ: Concentration-time profile of phenytoin after admixture with small volumes of intravenous fluids. *Am J Hosp Pharm* 1978;34:313-318.

9. Cranford RE, Leppik IE, Patrick B, et al: Intravenous phenytoin: clinical and pharmacokinetic aspects. *Neurology* 1978;28:874-880.

10. Leppik IE, Boucher BA, Wilder BJ, et al: Pharmacokinetics and safety of phenytoin prodrug given IV or IM in patients. *Neurology* 1990;40:456-460.

11. Lowenstein DH, Aminoff MJ, Simon RP: Barbiturate anesthesia in the treatment of status epilepticus. *Neurology* 1988;38:395-400.

12. Treiman DM, Walton NY, Kendrick CW: A progressive sequence of electroencephalographic changes during generalized convulsive status epilepticus. *Epilepsy Res* 1990;5:49-60.

13. Rothner AD, Erenberg G: Status epilepticus. *Pediatr Clin North Am* 1980;27:593-602.

14. Lockman LA, Kriel R, Laske D, et al: Phenobarbital dose for control of neonatal seizures. *Neurology* 1979;29: 1445-1449.

Chapter 13

Intractable Epilepsy and Surgical Management

Surgery has begun to play a larger role in the treatment of epilepsy. The advent of improved drug therapy has contributed to the rising use of surgery because it is now possible to rapidly maximize a patient's drug treatment, using blood levels to assess optimal treatment. Epilepsy should be controlled as soon as possible after its onset. Animal studies have shown that seizures may cause changes within the brain that may increase the probability of further seizures. Also, the social and emotional consequences of further seizures can be serious: loss of job, loss of driving privileges, and depression.

Patients are considered to have intractable epilepsy when their seizures have not been brought under complete control within 1 year after appropriate therapy has been started and documented with blood levels.[1] Table 1 lists the diagnostic codes for various seizure types. Because the severity of epilepsy varies among patients, use of the codes in Table 1 may help in correctly classifying patients with epilepsy. Once a patient has been found to have intractable epilepsy, a review of the case should be requested from a specialist familiar with the current presurgical evaluation. A preliminary assessment of the options for surgery can often be made from outpatient reveiw of the etiology and surface EEG readings. This may lead to further presurgical evaluation, including video-EEG monitoring (Table 1).[1]

Improved diagnostic techniques of video-EEG monitoring to localize the onset of seizures and improved imaging technology using magnetic resonance imaging (MRI) to detect lesions such as mesial temporal sclerosis have made the identification of potential surgical candidates more accurate and rapid.

Four types of surgery are available: removal of one lobe, usually the temporal lobe (temporal lobectomy); removal of cortex (topectomy); removal of a hemisphere (hemispherectomy); and sepa-

Table 1
ICD-9-CM Diagnostic Codes for Epilepsy

Diagnosis	Intractable	Not intractable
Generalized convulsive epilepsy	345.11	345.10
Partial epilepsy, with impairment of consciousness	345.41	345.40
Partial epilepsy, without mention of impairment of consciousness	345.51	345.50
Other forms of epilepsy	345.81	345.80
Epilepsy unspecified	345.91	345.90

ration of the two hemispheres by cutting the corpus callosum. By far the most widely performed surgery for epilepsy is temporal lobectomy. This is very successful in patients who have a specific epilepsy syndrome of mesial temporal sclerosis. Although success rates vary from center to center, complete control of seizures has been reported in up to 75% of cases, and worthwhile improvement in up to 90%.[2] More difficult is the removal of some portion of cortex; often, intracranial recording is required before surgery to achieve precise localization of the epileptogenic region and areas of "eloquent cortex," which cannot be removed without causing damage.

Hemispherectomy is reserved for a few patients with severe damage to one hemisphere with the presence of a relatively normal contralateral hemisphere. Corpus callosotomy is useful in patients with multifocal damage with rapid spread of seizure activity from one hemisphere to the other. Although surgery is increasing, there is little likelihood that this option will be useful for most patients with epilepsy. Nevertheless, an evaluation directed at establishing the appropriateness for surgery should be done for any patient whose seizures have not come under complete control.

History of Surgery

Surgery for epilepsy had its origin after World War I in Germany when interest developed in the surgical removal of posttraumatic scar tissue. At that time, local anesthesia was advanced enough to allow brain surgery on the awake patient. This was important because it permitted direct cortical recording and stimulation to identify the epileptic focus as well as areas of eloquent cortex. Wilder Penfield, Herbert Jasper, and their colleagues at the Montreal Neurological Institute began a long series of surgeries for epilepsy in 1934. This culminated in their classic book, *Epilepsy and the Functional Anatomy of the Brain.*[3] This described almost two decades of fastidious work analyzing numerous patients who had undergone recording and stimulation of the brain to identify epileptic regions. This book remains one of the more fascinating works in neurology because it describes in detail the responses to stimulation of various areas of the brain and because it builds the basis for much of our current understanding of regional brain function. Surgery for epilepsy remained limited until the last decade, when great improvements in diagnosis and surgical techniques made surgery available to a large number of patients with intractable epilepsy.[4,5]

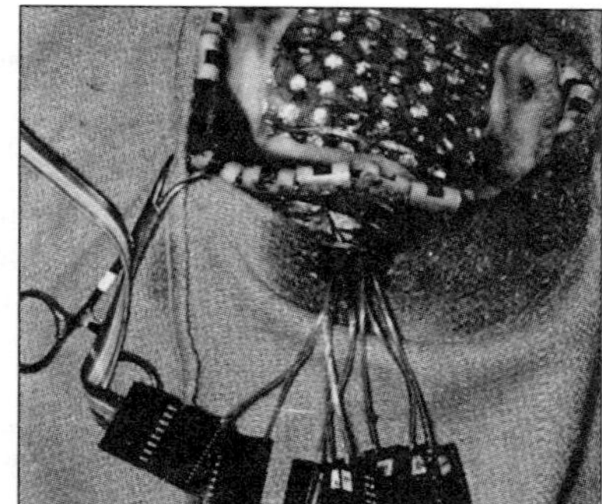

***Figure 1**—Placement of subdural grid for recording from the brain to locate onset of seizures. This grid consists of 64 contact points. Stimulation is performed to map out the motor and speech areas.*

Presurgical Evaluation

The most important element in successful outcome of surgery is accurate identification of the origin of the seizure. A critical development has been the use of inpatient video-EEG recording of seizures. Patients with intractable epilepsy are admitted to special units in which their antiepileptic medications are withdrawn, while they are monitored around the clock with EEG recording. Special electrodes, such as sphenoidal electrodes inserted through the masseter muscle to the foramen ovale, can be used to record from medial temporal lobes.

Neuropsychological testing is crucial in helping identify local areas of dysfunction. For example, deficits in verbal memory implicate the left temporal lobe. Because temporal lobectomy should be avoided if the remaining temporal lobe cannot maintain memory function, the intracarotid amytal test (Wada test) is critical.[6] During this test, first one and then the other carotid artery is injected with amytal, resulting in arrest of cerebral function of the injected area. Speech and memory testing is performed, and one is thus able to determine the approximate functional capacity of the opposite hemisphere in the absence of the injected hemisphere, providing an assessment of postoperative functioning.

MRI has become an important diagnostic tool. The new 1.5 to 2.0 Tesla MRI makes it possible to detect subtle hippocampal atrophy and mesial temporal sclerosis. If all four tests give congruent evidence of unilateral temporal involvement—surface EEG, neuropsychologic testing, MRI, and Wada—it may not be necessary to perform additional tests before surgery. However, if there is suggestion of bitemporal involvement, depth electrodes may be needed. In the past, almost all patients underwent depth electrode recordings prior to surgery. Positron emission tomography (PET scans) are useful in identifying focal areas of brain hypometabolism and may provide additional localizing and lateralizing information. A new development is the use of very-high-tesla MRI units for functional mapping of the brain.

Patients with frontal, parietal, and occipital lobe epilepsy are also potential surgical candidates. In these cases, however, cortical mapping before surgery may be necessary. Today, this can be done by implanting subdural grids from which stimulation and recording can be done to map the brain, much as was done by Penfield, but with the advantage of much longer recording and stimulating periods. The subdural grids may be used for 1 or 2 weeks before surgery (Figure 1). These grids are necessary in patients who have seizures emanating from the posterior part of the brain's temporal lobe in the speech-dominant hemisphere or in those where the origin is close to the motor strip.

Most surgery for epilepsy is done in the temporal lobe. However, many patients with intractable epilepsy are not good surgical candidates because of bitemporal or extratemporal foci. Some of these may be approached after grid mapping but, generally, complete remission of seizures is not as favorable, with 50% or less complete cure rates.

Some patients develop severe unihemispheral disorders, such as Rasmussen's encephalitis. Hemispherectomy may be quite helpful for these cases.[7] In patients with multifocal epilepsy with rapid generalization, cutting the corpus callosum can be useful for "drop" seizures in which patients suddenly fall to the floor, often sustaining major injuries. However, partial seizures may remain unaffected.[8]

References

1. Leppik IE: Intractable epilepsy in adults. In: Theodore WH, ed. *Surgical Treatment of Epilepsy* (*Epilepsy Res* suppl 5), 1992, pp 7-11.

2. King DW, Flanigin HF, Gallagher BB, et al: Temporal lobectomy for partial seizures: Evaluation, results, and a 1-year follow-up. *Neurology* 1986; 36:334-339.

3. Penfield W, Jasper H: *Epilepsy and the Functional Anatomy of the Human Brain.* Boston, Little, Brown and Co, 1954.

4. Luders HO: *Epilepsy Surgery.* New York, Raven Press, 1992.

5. Engel J Jr: *Surgical Treatment of the Epilepsies.* 2nd ed. New York, NY, Raven Press, 1993.

6. Wada J, Rasmussen T: Intracarotid injection of sodium amytal for the lateralization of cerebral speech dominance: Experimental and clinical observations. *J Neurosurg* 1960;17:266-282.

7. Rasmussen T: Hemispherectomy for seizures revisited. *Can J Neurol Sci* 1983;10:71-78.

8. Wyllie E: Corpus callosotomy for intractable generalized epilepsy. *J Pediatr* 1988; 113:255-261.

Chapter 14

Driving and Regulatory Issues

Physicians often become involved in regulatory issues when caring for patients with epilepsy because these may require medical information for resolution. A common area of physician involvement is certification of driving privileges. In addition, the recently enacted Americans with Disabilities Act has greatly increased the opportunities for patients with epilepsy and other medical problems to challenge restrictions and they will need medical reports to support their claims.

In the United States, laws and regulations emanate from federal, state, or local government. Those derived from federal government are enacted by Congress and are applicable to all of the states. These usually cover broad, national issues such as civil rights, Social Security, and Medicare. Areas such as driving restrictions and workmen's compensation are in the states' jurisdiction

Table 1
Legal and Regulatory Issues Involving Patients With Epilepsy

Federal
- Federal benefits (Social Security, Medicare and Medicaid)
- Military service (VA benefits)
- Americans With Disabilities Act

State
- Driving
- Employment (vocational rehabilitation)
- Family law (adoption, child custody)
- Workmen's compensation
- Criminal justice
- Access to health care

Table 1 lists areas of law and regulation by federal and state jurisdictions.

Driver Licensing

Every state regulates driver's license eligibility. These often include specific standards for persons with medical conditions.

In the case of seizure disorders, a physician becomes involved at two points: at the time of onset of seizures and at recertification of a patient with established epilepsy.

Each state has its own regulations regarding relicensing. Table 2 gives a summary of the key points. These regulations are subject to change, however, so a physician must become aware of the specific requirements in his or her state. The area of greatest change in the last few years has been the seizure-free period. In the past, most states required a 1-year period from the time of the last seizure. But because of the increasing recognition that patients with epilepsy do not differ significantly in overall driving safety from the general population, many states are liberalizing the requirements by shortening the time from the last seizure to restitution of driving privileges. Some states have removed the terms seizure or epilepsy from their statutes, and refer instead to episodes of loss of consciousness or control. Thus, conditions other than epilepsy are included in the regulations by implication. Some states also have medical review boards that will grant exceptions to the general rules. Some of these exceptions are:

- a breakthrough seizure caused by a physician-directed change in medication;
- an isolated seizure where the medical examination indicates that another seizure appears unlikely;
- a seizure related to a temporary illness;
- an established pattern of only nocturnal seizures;
- an established pattern of seizures that do not impair driving ability, ie, simple partial seizures with no loss of consciousness or control.

At the federal level, the United States Department of Transportation has regulations that bar anyone with any history of epilepsy from being licensed to drive in interstate trucking.

One area of uncertainty is the action to be taken after a single seizure. Most states require a diagnosis of epilepsy before the regulations regarding driving go into effect.

Table 2
Laws by State Relating to Driving and Epilepsy*

State	Seizure-Free Period	Physician Reporting
Alabama	1 year	No
Alaska	6 months	No
Arizona	1 year, with exceptions	No
Arkansas	1 year	No
California	**3, 6, or 12 months with exceptions**	**Yes**
Colorado	No set seizure-free period	No
Connecticut	No set seizure-free period	No
Delaware	**No set seizure-free period**	**Yes**
District of Columbia	1 year, with exceptions	No
Florida	6 months, with exceptions	No
Georgia	1 year; less if only nocturnal seizures	No
Hawaii	1 year, with exceptions	No
Idaho	1 year; 6 months with strong recommendation from doctor	No
Illinois	No set seizure-free period	No
Indiana	No set seizure-free period	No
Iowa	6 months; less if seizures nocturnal	No
Kansas	6 months	No
Kentucky	90 days	No
**Louisiana	1 year, with exceptions	No
Maine	6 months or longer	No
Maryland	90 days	No
Massachusetts	6 months	No
Michigan	6 months; less at discretion of department	No
Minnesota	6 months, with exceptions	No
**Mississippi	1 year	No
**Missouri	1 year	No
+Montana	6 months	No
+Nebraska	1 year, with exceptions	No

Nevada	**3 months, with exceptions**	**Yes**
+New Hampshire	1 year, less at discretion of department	No
New Jersey	**1 year; less on recommendation of Neurological Disorder Committee**	**Yes**
New Mexico	1 year	No
New York	1 year, with exceptions	No
North Carolina	1 year, with exceptions	No
North Dakota	1 year; restricted licenses available after 6 months	No
Ohio	No set seizure-free period	No
Oklahoma	1 year, with exceptions	No
Oregon	**6 months, with exceptions**	**Yes**
Pennsylvania	**6 months, with exceptions**	**Yes**
Puerto Rico	No set seizure-free period	No
Rhode Island	18 months; less at the discretion of Dept. of Transportation	No
South Carolina	6 months	No
**South Dakota	12 months; less with doctor's recommendation	No
Tennessee	6 months	No
**Texas	6 months with doctor's recommendation, with exceptions	No
Utah	3 months	No
Vermont	2 years, or 6 months with doctor's recommendation	No
Virginia	6 months, with exceptions	No
Washington	6 months	No
West Virginia	1 year, with exceptions	No
Wisconsin	3 months	No
Wyoming	1 year, with exceptions	No

* Modified from Epilepsy Foundation of America's Legal Advocacy Department and reflects data as of November 1995. Most states do not require physicians to report epilepsy.

** No appeal of license denial

\+ No periodic medical updates required

However, adults with a single seizure are at higher risk than the rest of the population for having a second seizure, as described in Chapter 4. Should a person have his or her driving restricted after a single seizure? This question does not have a simple answer. One must balance the small probability of a second seizure occurring while driving against the considerable loss of income, freedom, and self-esteem experienced by someone losing his or her driver's license. Unfortunately, the physician is caught in the middle of this difficult decision, and regardless of the action taken, in some cases the outcome will not be favorable.

In most states, the patient has the responsibility to report to the state the development of epilepsy or the occurrence of a seizure. In these states, the physician must counsel patients on their responsibilities, and document on the medical record that this has been done. This preserves the confidentiality of the physician-patient relationship and patients can freely discuss their condition.

However, six states—California, Delaware, Nevada, New Jersey, Oregon, and Pennsylvania—have mandatory physician-reporting requirements. While the exact terms of these provisions vary, they generally require any physician who diagnoses or treats a patient with epilepsy to report that patient's name, age, and address to a state agency, usually the department of motor vehicles or the department of public safety.

Most physicians feel that mandatory reporting laws may be counterproductive because they erode the confidential nature of the physician-patient relationship. Proper diagnosis and treatment of epilepsy depend greatly on the development of an honest, trusting relationship between a patient and his or her physician. Accurate information concerning seizure activity is critically important. If patients know or fear that their doctors are obligated to report their seizures to the state, those patients may withhold crucial information to avoid state sanctions. That nondisclosure of essential information could be fraught with serious medical consequences to the patient. One study showed that if patients know their physicians would report them, many would not inform their physicians of seizures they had had.[2]

Tort law in many states has recognized that physicians may be held liable for damages arising from the acts of their patients. Specifically, if a physician fails to instruct a patient about the risks associated with impairment from illness or medication, and a motor vehicle accident occurs because of the patient's compromised functioning, the physician may be held liable for some or all of the damages.[3]

The Epilepsy Foundation of America reviews legal issues and laws concerning persons with epilepsy. Its summary of these concerns provides an easy to understand overview of current court decisions and legislation.[4]

References

1. Hansotia P, Broste SK: The effect of epilepsy or diabetes mellitus on the risk of automobile accidents. *N Engl J Med* 1991;324:22-26.

2. Salinsky MC, Wegener K, Sinnema F: Epilepsy, driving laws, and patient disclosure to physicians. *Epilepsia* 1992; 33(3):472.

3. Freese v Lemmon, Iowa, 1973.

4. The legal rights of persons with epilepsy. An overview of legal issues and laws affecting persons with epilepsy. 6th ed. Maryland, Epilepsy Foundation of America, 1992.

Chapter 15

Quality of Life Issues

Seizures and the control of seizures engage only a small part of the daily life of a person with epilepsy. Most patients with epilepsy are otherwise normal, with the exception of having a propensity toward seizures. In many cases, seizures are infrequent, perhaps occurring only once every few months or even years. Between seizures, these persons have the potential to lead normal lives and be contributing members of society. However, the triple problem of medication side effects, personal fear of losing control, and society's revulsion of seeing a person struggle with a seizure add up to significant social barriers for the person with epilepsy (Table 1).

Table 1

Quality of Life Issues for Persons With Epilepsy

- Employment
- Driving
- Sports
- Cognition
- Personal safety

Employment

Although patients with epilepsy may have average or above-average intelligence, and otherwise be in good health, the unpredictable loss of consciousness can make them unsuitable for some jobs. While there are no hard-and-fast rules, clinicians generally agree that persons with epilepsy should avoid workplaces in which a sudden loss of consciousness may expose them or their coworkers to risk or injury.

Most obvious are jobs that require operation of motor vehicles. A person with a history of epilepsy cannot operate interstate trucks, even if seizures are controlled. Also, there are strict regulations applicable to persons with epilepsy who want to operate aircraft. At one time, the United States Air Force required all pilots to undergo EEG examinations and prohibited flight duty even for those who never had clinical seizures but who did have abnormal EEGs. Driving a forklift in a warehouse may also be contraindicated for some persons. However, if the seizures are well controlled, or if the epilepsy is in remission (such as after surgery), some of these jobs may be appropriate.

Another issue is working in heights. With proper safety equipment such as harnesses, which ideally should be available for all workers, the risk of injury with seizures is greatly diminished. Thus, working in high places should not be automatically excluded. The same applies to operating heavy equipment; with proper safety devices, this should not be a problem. If a person with epilepsy works on a farm, tractors should be equipped with a "dead-man" brake, a common device developed decades ago for train engineers, which shuts down the equipment when active control is lost.

There are very few office positions that should be denied a person with epilepsy. However, there may be some understandable reluctance to hire someone with epilepsy to work in a position that requires him or her to make a good impression with the public. One of my patients had relatively brief complex partial seizures that might not have been a problem for most persons, but he found them understandably disabling in his occupation as a funeral director. Thus, each person must have his or her needs assessed. Seizures in some situations may not pose a problem, whereas in others they would. A physician must evaluate each seizure type and frequency in relation to the demands of a specific job.

Often, employers who are at risk for lawsuits arising from workplace injuries may be overly conservative with restrictions against workers with epilepsy. Many states, however, have specific regulations protecting employers from excessive liability if an injury occurs in the workplace. On the other hand, the physician should be aware that there may be other factors that lead to an employer's discontent, such as poor work habits or poor interpersonal relationships, and epilepsy is used as the excuse. I have many patients who have frequent seizures in the workplace, but are deemed valuable employees because of their excellent work habits. In fact, their supervisors go to great lengths to make it possible for them to continue working.

Persons with epilepsy often

Table 2

Sports and Epilepsy

Permitted Sports (no restrictions)

aerobics	curling	jogging
archery	dancing	lacrosse
badminton	dogsledding	orienteering
ballet	discus throwing	shot-putting
baseball	fencing	soccer
basketball	field hockey	table tennis
bowling	high jumping	volleyball
broad jumping	fishing	weight lifting
cricket	gymnastics	wrestling
croquet	golfing	
cross-country skiing	hiking	

Possible Sports (reasonable precautions)

bicycling	ice skating	skiing (downhill)
bobsledding	kayaking	sledding
canoeing	mountain climbing	snowmobiling
diving	pole-vaulting	swimming
football	roller blading	tennis
horseback riding	rugby	water polo
hockey	sailing	
hunting	skating	

Prohibited Sports

boxing	polo	scuba diving
bungee jumping	rock climbing	skydiving
hang gliding	sailboarding	snorkeling
jousting	surfing	waterskiing

need help in securing appropriate employment, such as instructions on how to prepare a job application or how to prepare for an interview. Even when seizures are not severe or are unlikely to have much impact on the work, listing epilepsy on a job application might exclude a person from further consideration. In addition to governmental agencies, the local volunteer affiliates of the Epilepsy Foundation of America (4351 Garden City Drive, Landover, MD 20785) may have a training and placement program that can assist in finding work.

Fortunately, attitudes of employers have generally become more favorable towards persons with epilepsy over the last 30 years.[1] Nevertheless, persons with epilepsy may face employment problems, especially if they have had seizures while at work.

Sports

Participation in sports is popular for many persons in all ages of life. This is particularly the case for persons in school, where being on a team can be a major learning experience. Unfortunately, many parents and school officials use the excuse of preventing injury to unnecessarily limit epileptic students' participation in sports. This need not be the case (Table 2). A number of successful athletes have epilepsy. One example is Gary Howatt, a professional hockey player who has been an Epilepsy Foundation of America advocate for persons with epilepsy participating in sports. There is little or no evidence that physical fatigue, such as experienced in strenuous activity, will lead to a seizure. Indeed, one person with epilepsy runs marathon races and has never had a seizure while competing.

Common sense should prevail in choosing sporting activities in which to participate. In general, activities that involve the possibility of significant metabolic imbalances, such as scuba diving or very high-altitude mountain climbing, should be avoided. Also, sports that involve potential for serious injury from the loss of consciousness should be avoided. These include sports in which the body does not have contact with the ground, such as skydiving. Also, sports that carry a high risk for head injury should be avoided. Location and surroundings also play a role. Swimming, if done in a well-lighted pool with lifeguards and other persons aware of the swimmer's epilepsy, is not contraindicated. On the other hand, swimming in a river or lake should be prohibited. Some years ago, the American Medical Association's Committee on Medical Aspects of Sports published the following statement: "There is ample evidence that patients with epilepsy will not be affected by indulging in any sport, including football, provided the normal safeguards

Table 3

First Aid for Seizures

Generalized tonic-clonic seizures

The patient may have a warning, cry out, stiffen, fall, and then rhythmically jerk arms and legs. These movements are very strong and cannot be stopped.

At the onset or during the seizure:

- Help the patient into a prone position
- Remove eyeglasses
- Clear area of harmful objects
- Loosen tight clothing around neck
- Do not restrain the patient
- Do not force any object into the patient's mouth

After the seizure:

- Turn the patient to one side to permit mouth to drain
- Continue to observe the patient until fully awake

If the patient is known to have epilepsy, it is not necessary to call for medical help unless:

- An injury has occurred
- Seizures do not stop in 2 to 3 minutes
- A second seizure occurs
- The person requests an ambulance

Complex partial seizures

The patient may stare without focusing, not speak, perform aimless movements, smack lips or appear to chew, fidget with clothes. Sometimes this behavior resembles that of a drunk or drugged person.

During the seizure:

- Do not try to stop or restrain patient
- Guide the patient gently away from harmful objects

After the seizure:

- Stay with the patient until fully alert
- Reassure others that this behavior was medically caused

for sports participation are followed, including adequate head protection."[2]

Sexuality and Interpersonal Relations

With the exception of barbiturates or benzodiazepines, antiepileptic drugs (AEDs) do not appear to have a major effect on libido. Although AEDs may have a minor effect on some hormones, including estrogen and testosterone, these changes are generally small. With proper counseling, most persons with epilepsy can have normal sexual relations.[3]

The psychological issues of low self-esteem and poorly developed interpersonal skills account for greater limitations. Unfortunately, many children with epilepsy are socially ostracized in school. Parents may be overprotective. Siblings may be unsupportive. The fear of loss of control during a date is very frightening. Lack of a driving license is a major limitation. Despite these issues, many persons with epilepsy overcome barriers and develop stable personal relationships, marry, and have families. Women with epilepsy and their offspring are at higher risk for complications (Chapter 11) but most are able to have normal families. Breastfeeding is not contraindicated; the Physician's Desk Reference® includes a prohibition on breast-feeding for any mother who is taking an AED because such drugs are present in breast milk. But this prohibition seems unwarranted because infants are exposed to much higher drug levels in utero.

Personal Safety

A person with epilepsy lives with the constant fear that seizures may strike at any moment. One survey showed more than 60% of persons with epilepsy feared dying during a seizure. Yet, very few persons die during a seizure. Thus, physicians often do not address this topic, or, if they do, discuss the statistics rather than focusing on the emotional aspects of the question. Persons with epilepsy also fear injury. This fear is justified because most generalized tonic-clonic seizures can be associated with injury. During complex partial seizures, patients may scald themselves with hot tap water, set clothes on fire from gas stoves, fall in the shower, drown in the bathtub, etc. Severe burns from irons, stoves, and other household items may occur.[4] A physician should be sensitive to these fears, and be willing to counsel the patient in common sense safety issues. Occupational therapists are useful professionals to help in this area.

Persons with epilepsy need to be able to instruct their families, friends, and coworkers in what to do in case of a seizure. Placing objects into the mouth of a person stricken with a seizure is no longer considered an appropriate intervention because teeth may be broken, oral tissues damaged, or the gag reflex triggered. This last consequence may lead to vomiting and the possibility of aspiration pneumonia. Also, it may obstruct the airway, decreasing the effectiveness of the marked respiratory effort that often follows a seizure (Table 3).

Driving

Of all the limitations placed on a person with epilepsy, loss of driving privilege may be the most serious. Not being permitted to drive drastically alters a person's mobility and suddenly puts him or her in a dependent role. This loss may be particularly devastating to active, independent persons living in areas lacking adequate public transportation. One of my patients confessed that the diagnosis of having a brain tumor was not nearly as devastating as losing driving privileges. The medico-legal aspects of this topic are covered in Chapter 14.

Cognition

All major AEDs have some effect on cognition. These effects are usually mild, and usually do not worsen with chronic treatment.[5] Some persons, especially those with inquisitive, active minds, will describe difficulties with memory, lethargy, decreased rapidity of calculations, and other effects. Although many of these effects cannot be measured readily, patients' reports of them must be appreciated. Sometimes these effects can be more troubling than the seizures, especially if the seizures are simple partial events. Therefore, a physician must evaluate the severity of each seizure type, and weigh it against the cost of side effects. Simple partial seizures can rarely be completely controlled with medication, but they do not interfere with consciousness or function and thus do not need to be eliminated. Effective treatment involves participation of the person with epilepsy in the treatment team. For the best outcome, a physician should be able to provide a comprehensive treatment program involving many professionals in the team.[6] Surgery for epilepsy is best done in a team setting, because many patients will continue to have psychosocial problems even after temporal lobectomy.[7]

Epilepsy can affect anyone at any time. In my practice I

treat a number of professionals who developed epilepsy after making a considerable investment in careers and lifestyles. The disorder forces them to deal with profound changes in their lives. Below are brief case descriptions of patients who have developed epilepsy and are attempting resolution of complex issues.

Case 1. A second-year medical student had a single generalized tonic-clonic seizure after sleep deprivation. His wife witnessed the seizure. The EEG was normal, and treatment was not started. A year later, a second generalized tonic-clonic seizure occurred and clinicians uncovered an additional history of a family member with epilepsy. The medical student had been interested in a surgical subspecialty, and, after treatment was begun, his career was put back on track as the seizures were controlled. Some mild cognitive effects were noted initially; these cleared with change in medication and time. After successful completion of medical school, the patient entered residency training. However, because of interrupted sleep patterns and stressful work load, seizures began to occur a few times a year despite increasing doses of medication. Driving privileges and operating room activities were suspended. Fortunately, the patient's talents and personal qualities were such that he successfully completed a modified training program. Then, a practice routine was established in which call schedules and duties were adjusted to accommodate the possibility of seizures, which have subsequently come under much better control.

Case 2. A young woman had some brief events in college, which, in retrospect, were probably simple partial seizures. A tonic-clonic seizure occurred after she married a medical student. Evaluation was negative, and no further seizures occurred until her first pregnancy. All of the concerns regarding AEDs and fetal risk were reviewed, and a medication was started. She had no more generalized tonic-clonic seizures but she did have brief complex partial seizures a few times a year. These were not consequential and she was able to raise her family and participate in many community activities. During a subsequent pregnancy, AEDs were discontinued, and shortly thereafter a marked increase in seizures occurred. They were better controlled with the reinstitution of medicines. But after her delivery, seizures continued to worsen and she became profoundly depressed. A complete evaluation was performed, and seizures were found to be multifocal in origin, probably related to early childhood encephalopathy and not approachable by surgery. Because of concerns regarding her ability to care for her children (probably overstated) and her inability to drive, a nanny was hired to help care for the children and to serve as a chauffeur. The patient has developed an understandably high degree of frustration, and is in a counseling program and an epilepsy support program. Although she has approximately four complex partial seizures per month, and so is otherwise normal the other 25 days of the month, her life-style, self-image, and actions with her family have changed profoundly.

Case 3. A midcareer physician in a nonsurgical, clinical academic setting had a single seizure. After considerable research on the topic, it was decided to begin monotherapy with a standard AED. No seizures occurred until the patient attended a convention and realized he forgot the medication. He experienced a seizure that was observed by a few of his friends and colleagues. Medication was immediately restarted. He has been seizure-free for some years, but continues to take the medication. Rationally, this person knows that he is unlikely to have another seizure. But the fear of possibly having another seizure has created a constant level of anxiety, which is revealed only to the most trusted confidants.

Case 4. A suburban teenager developed mild viral encephalitis. Before this, he had been active in sports, was a good student, and had a gregarious, pleasant personality. A few months later, intractable seizures began. Despite trying a number of medications, including some in the testing phase, his seizures were not well controlled. He also experienced a decline in his intellectual functioning. He was able to finish high school and move into a group home for persons with epilepsy who had relatively normal functional capabilities. However, funding cutbacks forced this facility to close. Meanwhile, the patient's father had advanced his career and the family moved to a different city. More than 10 years after the onset of epilepsy, the patient is living in a sheltered group home with individuals of much lower functioning level.

These case histories illustrate that the development of epilepsy can have a profound impact on a person's life. However, with good care, the potential of achieving many goals can be met.

References

1. Hicks RA, Hicks MJ: Attitudes of major employers toward the employment of people with epilepsy: a 30-year study. *Epilepsa* 1991;32(1):86-88.

2. Corbitt RW: Epileptics and contact sports. *JAMA* 1974; 229:820-821.

3. Frazer C, Gumnit RJ: Sexuality and the person with epilepsy. In: Gumnit RJ, ed. *Living Well With Epilepsy*. New York, Demos Publications, 1990, pp 105-108.

4. Spitz M: Severe burns as a consequence of seizures in patients with epilepsy. *Epilepsia* 1992;33(1):103-107.

5. Dodrill CB, Wilensky AJ: Neuropsychological abilities before and after 5 years of stable antiepileptic drug therapy. *Epilepsia* 1992;33(2): 327-324.

6. Frazer C, Gumnit RJ: How to be an effective member of your health-care team. In: Gummit RJ, ed. *Living Well With Epilepsy*. New York, Demos Publications, 1990, pp 21-25.

7. Bladin PF: Psychosocial difficulties and outcome after temporal lobectomy. *Epilepsia* 1992;33(5):898-907.

Chapter 16

Comprehensive Treatment of a Person With Epilepsy

Providing the appropriate treatment for the person with epilepsy can be a rewarding challenge for a physician. Moreover, proper treatment of epilepsy can be one of the most cost-effective expenditures of resources because it can enable a person with epilepsy to be a fully productive citizen. Most persons with epilepsy do not have a progressive disorder and so can lead normal, productive lives. However, epilepsy is still a frightening diagnosis for a person to confront because of the disorder's negative image.

The Epilepsy Foundation of America (EFA) has commissioned opinion polls over the last decades that have shown some improvement in public attitudes but still many misconceptions about this disorder. But epilepsy does not need to be "horrible," as Aretaeus called it. With current treatments, seizures can be controlled in most patients. Moreover, improved diagnostic techniques can quickly identify those few patients with serious etiologies, and then point to appropriate therapy. Those patients with no significant central nervous system disease can be reassured.

In epilepsy, both medical and psychosocial issues must be treated. A person's seizures may come under complete control, but if issues of driving, employment, self-image, and personal interactions are not addressed, total reintegration is not possible.

Key Treatment Points

Let us recapitulate the key elements in the medical treatment of epilepsy:

- Correctly differentiate between epileptic seizures and nonepileptic seizures (cardiogenic, psychogenic), or other phenomena resembling seizures (syncope, etc).
- Classify seizure types.
- Classify epilepsy syndrome.
- Choose the most appropriate medication based on the seizure type and the medication's side effects, and start treatment with a single drug.
- Obtain blood before treatment for baseline hematologic

and hepatic parameters.

- Check blood levels of the chosen antiepileptic drug two or three times in the first 6 months of treatment to determine that target levels have been attained and are being maintained.
- If seizures are controlled and blood levels are adequate, monitor every 6 months of each year for the duration of treatment.
- If a person's seizures are not controlled with adequate doses and levels of the standard medications, refer the patient to a clinician who specializes in epilepsy for a second opinion. At this point, the diagnosis of epilepsy must be verified, combination therapy may be used, and evaluation of surgical options considered.

Here is a recapitulation of the key elements in the treatment of the psychosocial issues:

- Review the pertinent issues:

  1. attitude of the patient towards seizures

  2. attitude of spouse, parents, relatives, coworkers, teachers, and other key persons toward epilepsy

  3. need to drive
- Develop an educational plan to address the problem areas.
- Monitor progress in dealing with the social issues.

The medical issues can be dealt with effectively in a standard physician-patient interaction. But the psychosocial issues often require the involvement of other persons. Fortunately, much educational information has been developed by the EFA, which can be very helpful in providing educational and support materials (Epilepsy Foundation of America, 4351 Garden City Drive, Landover, Maryland, 20785, 800-EFA-1000). Many local EFA affiliates have offices across the United States and are listed in telephone directories. Their staff can often provide assistance through support groups for dealing with the emotional stresses of epilepsy.

Thus, by comprehensively addressing the issues faced by a person with epilepsy, treatment can, in many cases, lead to a favorable outcome.

Index

A

B

C

D

E

F

G

H

I

J

K

L

M

N

O

P

Q

R

S

T

U

V

W

Z

NOTES

NOTES

NOTES

NOTES

NOTES

NOTES